Minimally Invasive Glaucoma Surgery

Chelvin C. A. Sng • Keith Barton
Editors

Minimally Invasive Glaucoma Surgery

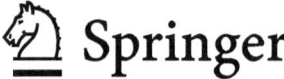 Springer

Editors
Chelvin C. A. Sng
National University Hospital
Singapore
Singapore

Keith Barton
Moorfields Eye Hospital
London
UK

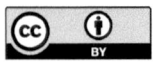

This book is an open access publication.
ISBN 978-981-15-5631-9   ISBN 978-981-15-5632-6   (eBook)
https://doi.org/10.1007/978-981-15-5632-6

This Springer imprint is published by the registered company Springer Nature Singapore Pte Ltd.
The registered company address is: 152 Beach Road, #21-01/04 Gateway East, Singapore 189721, Singapore

Foreword

The last decade has witnessed an explosion of novel therapies that have heralded the era of interventional glaucoma. Minimally invasive glaucoma surgery (MIGS) has been the center piece of this movement, providing ophthalmologists and patients with an alternative to topical medications or traditional conjunctival surgery. These procedures share a common approach to minimize normal anatomical and physiological disruption in an effort to reduce risks and hasten recovery and improve quality of life. While it remains to be seen what the impact of MIGS on reducing the global burden of glaucoma will be, this field has generated substantial interest in improving the outcomes of MIGS procedures.

With the vast array of MIGS options now available worldwide, there is a great need for a concise, easily accessible, and complete review of these procedures. Understanding the design, surgical technique variations, complications and management, and patient selection is essential for the successful incorporation of MIGS into clinical practice.

Edited by two well-respected internationally renowned glaucoma specialists, Chelvin Sng and Keith Barton, *Minimally Invasive Glaucoma Surgery* provides a comprehensive review of the field. A unique feature of this book is the global view of MIGS, with a wide international cast of experts contributing to this cutting-edge book. An overview and essential anatomy of the outflow pathways provides the reader with a firm basic foundation for MIGS as a starting point. One can then immerse oneself on a specific procedure with the latest techniques, evidence and results. MIGS procedures can be differentiated based on their outflow target (Schlemm's canal/conventional outflow, suprachoroidal/uveoscleral, and subconjunctival). *Minimally Invasive Glaucoma Surgery* covers each approach with the necessary breadth and depth to assist the beginner, intermediate and advanced surgeon. The book finishes with both controversies and a global view of MIGS discussed in a thought-provoking manner.

Sng and Barton have put together an excellent and comprehensive collection of topics on MIGS, authored by top global experts in the field. This book serves a great reference for those looking to better understand MIGS and the role it plays in glaucoma management.

Iqbal Ike K. Ahmed
Department of Ophthalmology
and Vision Sciences
University of Toronto
Toronto, ON, Canada

Contents

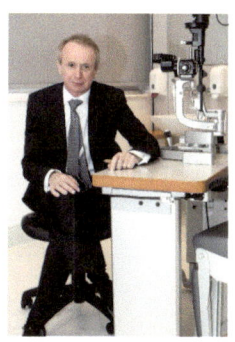

Keith Barton, MD, FRCP, FRCS, FRCOphth, is a consultant ophthalmologist and glaucoma specialist at Moorfields Eye Hospital, honorary reader in UCL Institute of Ophthalmology, co-chair of Ophthalmology Futures Forums, and editor-in-chief of the *British Journal of Ophthalmology*.

His areas of interest are the surgical management of glaucoma, especially surgical devices and secondary glaucomas and specifically the management of glaucoma in uveitis. He has been an investigator in the TVT study and PTVT study, co-chair of the Ahmed Baerveldt comparison study, and a member of the trial management committees of both the treatment of advanced glaucoma (TAGS) and lasers in glaucoma and ocular hypertension (LIGHT) studies (www.keithbarton.co.uk, https://uk.linkedin.com/in/keithbarton1, www.glaucoma-surgery.org).

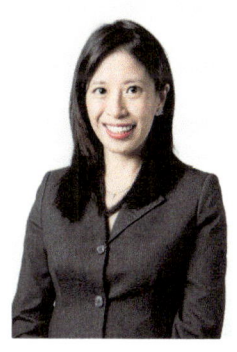

Chelvin C. A. Sng, MBBChir, MA, FRCSEd, is an associate professor and senior consultant at the National University Hospital in Singapore. She graduated from Gonville and Caius College in Cambridge University with triple first class honours and distinctions. As a recipient of the Academic Medicine and Development Award, she completed her glaucoma fellowship at Moorfields Eye Hospital. A/Prof Sng has a special interest in the use of glaucoma drainage devices and is amongst the first surgeons in Asia to be accredited in the use of several novel micro-invasive glaucoma surgery (MIGS) devices. She is also the co-inventor of the Paul Glaucoma Implant, which has attained CE mark and is currently undergoing commercialization. A/Prof Sng has received international awards from AAO, ASCRS, ANZGIG, APAO, and ARVO. She is the convenor of the Asia-Pacific Glaucoma Society (APGS)—MIGS Interest Group and the secretary of the Glaucoma Association of Singapore (GLAS).

Overview of MIGS

Jing Wang and Keith Barton

The term, minimally- or micro-invasive glaucoma surgery (MIGS), first coined around 2008 (II Ahmed, personal communication) has entered common ophthalmic parlance and is playing an increasing role in the management of glaucoma patients. In common, the devices and procedures referred to, are safer, less tissue invasive and associated with faster recovery than traditional filtering surgery, such as trabeculectomy or aqueous shunt implantation [1]. While the term initially referred only to *ab interno* Schlemm's canal bypass stents such as the iStent, it has expanded, though with somewhat inconsistent adoption, both by clinicians and by the manufacturers, not all of whom are enthusiastic about applying the MIGS label to their device, to encompass both *ab externo* and *ab interno* canal procedures, suprachoroidal implants, external filtration devices and to some degree, even new types of cyclodestruction. On the horizon are also drug-eluting implants. The US Food and Drug Administration (USFDA) defines MIGS as devices or procedures that lower intra-ocular pressure (IOP) with either an *ab interno* or *ab externo* approach, associated with little or no scleral dissection and minimal or no conjunctival manipulation, though USFDA workshops and guidance have tended to consider only implantable devices [2, 3]. This book covers the techniques that are most commonly regarded as eligible to sit under the MIGS umbrella, whether or not industry or clinicians prefer to call them MIGS. Others, such as the Ex-PRESS shunt (Alcon Laboratories, Inc., Fort Worth, Texas, USA), SOLX Gold Glaucoma Shunt (GGS, SOLX Ltd.,

J. Wang
Centre Universitaire d'ophtalmologie (CUO), Hôpital du Saint-Sacrement, CHU-Quebec, Québec, QC, Canada

Laval University, Québec, QC, Canada

K. Barton (✉)
Glaucoma Service, Moorfields Eye Hospital, London, UK

Institute of Ophthalmology, University College London, London, UK
e-mail: keith@keithbarton.co.uk

1
C. C. A. Sng, K. Barton (eds.), *Minimally Invasive Glaucoma Surgery*,
https://doi.org/10.1007/978-981-15-5632-6_1

Waltham, MA, USA) and canaloplasty have some similarities to MIGS techniques and devices, but will not be covered in detail.

A number of MIGS devices and techniques have relatively modest efficacy but, potential utility in a very large group of glaucoma patients with disease that is insufficiently severe to justify the invasiveness of conventional filtration surgery and the consequent intensity of postoperative care, yet burdened with medication and the attendant side effects and compliance issues thereof. A simple additional technique at the time of cataract surgery could have significant quality of life benefits for a large number of these patients. On the other hand, some MIGS devices can potentially achieve efficacy approaching that of traditional filtering surgery and are appropriate in selected individuals when larger IOP reductions are required, the exception being cases where glaucoma is very advanced.

Irrespective of the modest efficacy of many MIGS devices and techniques, the favourable safety profile lowers the threshold for early glaucoma surgery, especially when combined with cataract surgery, potentially delaying the requirement for more invasive surgery and associated risks. The additional reduction in the medication burden has the potential to reduce intolerance, improve quality of life and lower the long-term cost of medication while improving adherence.

MIGS can be categorized according to the tissue they target (or bypass): trabecular meshwork (TM) MIGS, subconjunctival MIGS, suprachoroidal MIGS and newer cycloablation procedures. MIGS devices include iStent Trabecular Micro-Bypass Stent and iStent *inject* (Glaukos Corporation, San Clemente, CA, USA), Hydrus Microstent (Ivantis Inc., Irvine, CA, USA), the XEN Gel Implant (Allergan plc, Dublin, Ireland) and PRESERFLO (formerly InnFocus) MicroShunt (Santen Pharmaceutical Co. Ltd., Osaka, Japan) (Table 1.1). At present, as a result of the

Table 1.1 Procedures and implants that fall broadly within the minimally invasive category of glaucoma surgery though a number of those listed would not be typically described as MIGS

Schlemm's canal	Subconjunctival	Suprachoroidal	Ciliary body coagulation
Stenting iStent Trabecular Micro-Bypass Stent iStent *inject* Hydrus Microstent	Xen Gel Implant PRESERFLO MicroShunt	iStent Supra MINIject (CyPass Micro-Stent)	High-Intensity Focused Ultrasound cyclocoagulation Micropulse diode laser cyclophotocoagulation Endocyclophotocoagulation
Cutting Trabectome (*Ab interno* trabeculotomy) Gonioscopy-assisted transluminal trabeculotomy (GATT) Excimer laser trabeculostomy Kahook Dual Blade (KDB)			
Dilating *Ab interno* canaloplasty (ABiC)			

withdrawal of the CyPass Micro-Stent (Alcon Laboratories, Inc., Fort Worth, Texas, USA), there are no commercially available devices that drain to the supra-choroidal space, though others are in development.

While there are a number of pathways targeted by MIGS devices, most MIGS procedures in which a device is not implanted, are designed to eliminate trabecular meshwork resistance from the outflow pathway: *ab interno* trabeculotomy (Trabectome; NeoMedix Corporation, San Juan Capistrano, CA, USA) and gonioscopic-assisted transluminal trabeculotomy (GATT). Newer surgical instruments such as the Kahook Dual Blade (New World Medical, Rancho Cucamonga, CA, USA) and TRAB360 (Sight Sciences Inc., Menlo Park, CA, USA) are designed for *ab interno* removal of TM tissue to enhance physiological TM outflow system.

Ab interno canaloplasty (ABiC, Ellex Medical Pty Ltd., Adelaide, Australia) differs slightly in that it primarily dilates Schlemm's canal, although a small cut is made through trabecular meshwork to access the canal.

Concurrent with the appearance of the MIGS genre, a number of new cycloablation procedures have also appeared including micropulse diode laser trans-scleral cyclophotocoagulation (MicroPulse P3, IRIDEX IQ810 Laser System, Mountain View, CA, USA), applied externally via a new type of probe and High-Intensity Focused Ultrasound cyclocoagulation (EyeOP1 HIFU, EyeTechCare, Rillieux-la-Pape, France), applied externally but delivering a metered dose of ultrasound energy to the ciliary body. Endocylophotocoagulation (ECP), which was developed in the late 1990s, is analogous to conventional diode laser CPC, but applied via an *ab interno* approach and could also be considered in this category.

1.1 Trabecular Meshwork MIGS Devices and Techniques

Trabecular meshwork (TM) MIGS procedures and devices are numerous. They aim to eliminate trabecular meshwork resistance in the normal physiological outflow pathway in patients with mild-to-moderate glaucoma and ocular hypertension (OHT). They are indicated in combination with cataract surgery. In patients with chronic primary angle closure, the TM outflow system has likely long-standing and irreversible damage; TM MIGS procedures or implants should be approached with caution as the drainage pathway created whether stent or trabeculotomy, may occlude with iris because of the narrow angle. In angle closure, these procedures should generally be considered only after cataract surgery and confirmation that the angle has widened sufficiently that the risk of occlusion is low. In patients with advanced glaucoma, where the maximum possible pressure lowering is often desirable in order to minimize the risk of disease progression, TM MIGS procedures are not ideal as there is an opportunity cost in not achieving IOP control with the first surgical procedure.

All TM MIGS procedures involve direct gonioscopic visualization during surgery. TM MIGS devices include iStent Trabecular Micro-Bypass Stent, iStent *inject* (Fig. 1.1) and Hydrus Microstent (Fig. 1.2) [4–6]. These three devices aim to enhance TM outflow by stenting the Schlemm's canal. iStent Trabecular Micro-Bypass Stent and iStent *inject* are manufactured from heparin-coated titanium.

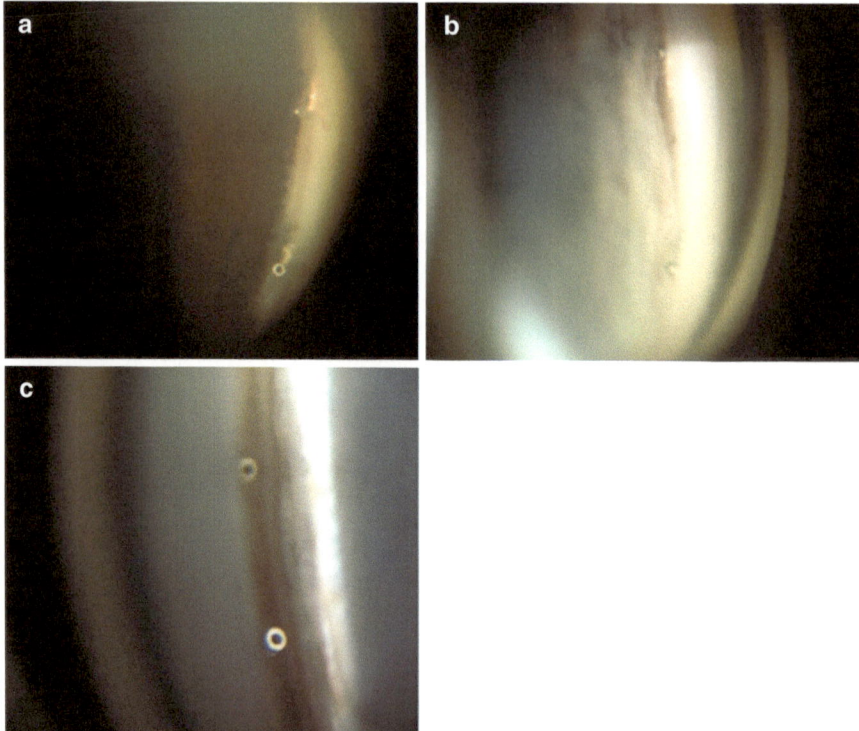

Fig. 1.1 Two iStent Trabecular Micro-Bypass Stents in the Schlemm's canal of two different patients (**a** and **b**) and two iStent *inject* implants in the trabecular meshwork (**c**). (Copyright Moorfields Eye Hospital and Keith Barton; reproduced with permission)

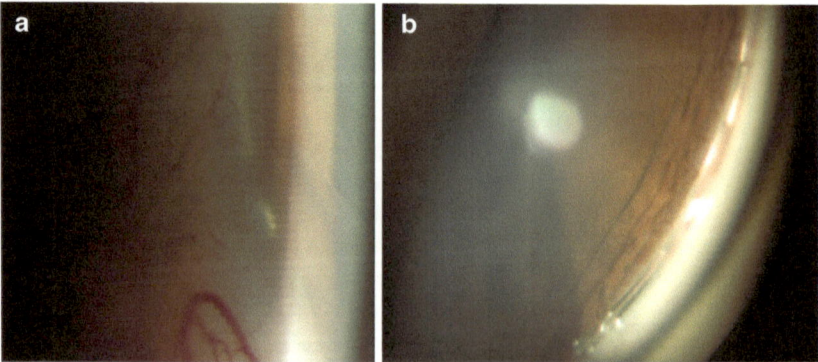

Fig. 1.2 The inlet of a Hydrus Microstent visible externally (**a**) and the Hydrus Microstent in the trabecular meshwork on gonioscopy (**b**). (Copyright Moorfields Eye Hospital and Keith Barton; reproduced with permission)

iStent Trabecular Micro-Bypass Stent is a 1 mm long, L-shaped device with a 120 μm lumen diameter. iStent *inject* is conically shaped, 360 μm in length and 230 μm at its largest diameter. The Hydrus Microstent is made of nitinol and is a crescent-shaped trabecular scaffold of 8 mm in length with a variable lumen diameter between 185 and 292 μm. Company-sponsored prospective randomized controlled trials have compared the effect of cataract surgery on IOP when combined with the iStent Trabecular Micro-Bypass Stent or the Hydrus Microstent to the effect of cataract surgery alone [4, 6]. Both demonstrated a modest but more sustained IOP-lowering effect in the group receiving cataract surgery combined with the TM MIGS device 2 years after surgery. All three are USFDA approved, at the time of writing, for implantation at the time of cataract extraction, but not for stand-alone surgery. In Europe, they are licensed for both.

Other TM procedures such as *ab interno* trabeculotomy (AIT) or Trabectome, GATT, Kahook Dual Blade and TRAB360 cut rather than stent the TM to varying degrees. Trabectome is the earliest FDA-approved TM removal procedure. It has a disposable 19.5-gauge handpiece with irrigation, aspiration and electrocautery combined. The tip of the Trabectome removes TM tissue and coagulates at the same time. Trabectome surgery is either performed at the beginning of cataract surgery or as a stand-alone procedure [7]. The Kahook Dual Blade is a disposable knife designed to remove a strip of TM tissue via a temporal incision. With a single incision, the Kahook Dual Blade and Trabectome can remove up to 120° of TM tissue, whereas GATT and TRAB360 (Sight Sciences, Menlo Park, CA, USA) can remove the entire TM tissue. GATT can be performed using either an illuminated micro-catheter (iTrack, Ellex Medical Pty Ltd., Adelaide, Australia)—designed originally for *ab externo* canaloplasty procedure—or a 5-0 polypropylene or Nylon suture [8]. Under direct gonioscopic view, a micro vitreoretinal (MVR) blade is used to incise the TM wall, after which the catheter or suture is advanced to cannulate Schlemm's canal through the incision. Complete 360° catheterization of Schlemm's canal may not be possible in all eyes. A prospective non-comparative case series has reported sustained IOP lowering for up to 2 years after GATT [9]. As 360° trabeculotomy becomes a popular first-line intervention in primary congenital glaucoma, there has been some interest in treating juvenile open-angle glaucoma with GATT as a primary surgical option.

1.2   Subconjunctival MIGS Devices

The XEN Gel Implant (Allergan; formerly known as XEN Gel Stent, AqueSys Inc.) (Fig. 1.3) and PRESERFLO (formerly InnFocus) MicroShunt (Santen Pharmaceutical Co. Ltd.) (Fig. 1.4) are the two currently available subconjunctival MIGS devices [10, 11]. The XEN Gel Implant is a soft porcine-derived collagen implant that is inserted, *ab interno*, from the anterior chamber to subconjunctival space. Six millimetres long and with an internal diameter of 45 μm, the XEN is preloaded in an injector. Its major potential advantage over traditional filtering

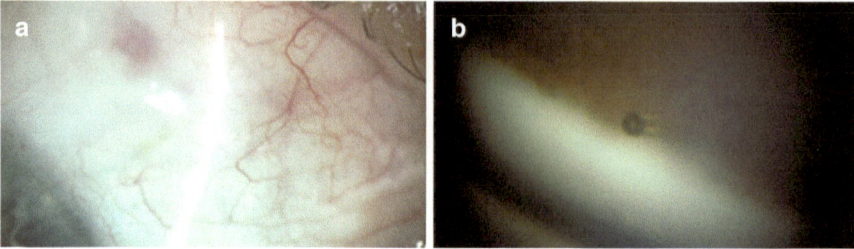

Fig. 1.3 XEN Gel Implant visible under the conjunctiva with a diffuse overlying drainage bleb (**a**) and the XEN Gel Implant visible in the anterior chamber (**b**). (Copyright Moorfields Eye Hospital and Keith Barton; reproduced with permission)

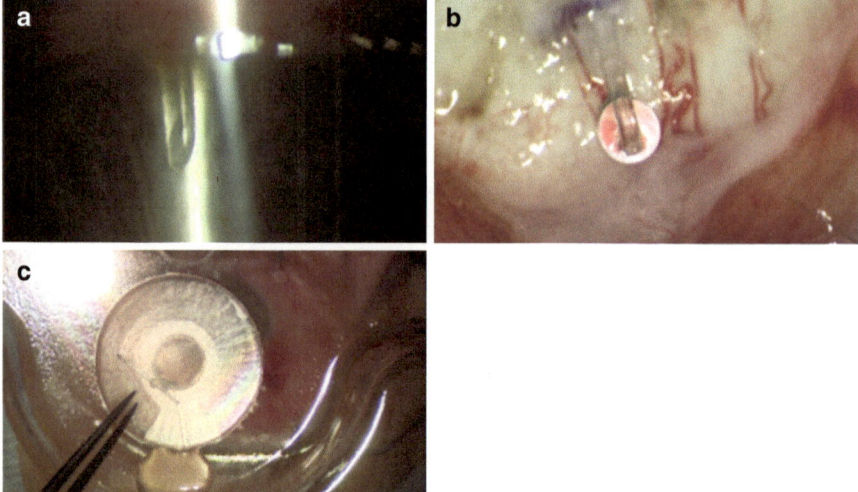

Fig. 1.4 The PRESERFLO MicroShunt in the anterior chamber (**a**), an external view showing aqueous drainage during implantation and before conjunctival closure (**b**) and the device prior to implantation (**c**). (Copyright Moorfields Eye Hospital and Keith Barton; reproduced with permission)

surgery is the avoidance of a conjunctival incision. However, the lack of conjunctival dissection requires precise placement of the XEN under the conjunctival tissue as the lumen of the XEN is easily blocked by Tenon's capsule. This explains a significantly higher rate of needling with the XEN [12]. Similar to the XEN Gel Implant, the PRESERFLO MicroShunt is also a tube that diverts aqueous humour from the anterior chamber to the subconjunctival space. The MicroShunt differs from the XEN in that it is implanted via an *ab externo* approach, necessitating conjunctival dissection. Unlike the XEN, the MicroShunt is of purely synthetic construction—poly(styrene-*block*-isobutylene-*block*-styrene) or SIBS. A randomized controlled trial comparing the MicroShunt with mitomycin C (MMC) to trabeculectomy with MMC for primary open angle glaucoma (POAG) is currently ongoing

(ClinicalTrial: NCT01881425). This is currently the only MIGS device that has been compared to trabeculectomy in a randomized clinical trial.

The IOP-lowering efficacy of subconjunctival MIGS, in selected cases, appears to approach that of traditional filtering surgery, thereby offering the possibility that they might have utility in more advanced or normal pressure glaucoma. On the other hand, subconjunctival MIGS are bleb-forming procedures and serious bleb-related complications such as infection, leakage and implant exposure have been reported [13].

1.3 Suprachoroidal MIGS Devices

Until recently, CyPass Micro-Stent was the only available suprachoroidal MIGS. It is a fenestrated micro-stent of 6.35 mm long with an external diameter of 510 µm and an internal diameter of 300 µm. It is made of a biocompatible polyamide material. The COMPASS trial is a randomized controlled trial comparing the effect of combined cataract surgery and CyPass insertion to cataract surgery alone in 505 POAG patients [14]. Two years after surgery, the IOP was lower on less medication in the group that underwent combined CyPass Micro-Stent implantation and cataract surgery than those that had cataract surgery alone. A prospective series of CyPass Micro-Stent implantation as a solo procedure in POAG patients with uncontrolled IOP demonstrated effective IOP lowering and avoided conventional filtering procedures in 83% of patients at 1 year follow-up [15]. After the COMPASS study was extended to 5 years after surgery (COMPASS XT), there was a significantly higher rate of endothelial cell loss in the combined CyPass Micro-Stent and cataract group compared to the cataract group alone. For this reason, the manufacturer (Alcon Laboratories, Inc., Fort Worth, Texas, USA) voluntarily withdrew the CyPass Micro-Stent from the market in August 2018, although it is estimated that there are currently around 33,000 implanted CyPass Micro-Stents in the world and managing the risk of endothelial loss may be an ongoing concern for several years after the withdrawal [16].

The iStent Supra (Glaukos) is a suprachoroidal stent made of polyethersulfone and heparin-coated titanium with a lumen diameter of 165 µm. The iStent Supra is not commercially available and there have been no prospective published efficacy studies at the time of writing.

1.4 Cyclophotocoagulation (CPC) Procedures

Cyclophotocoagulation procedures are also minimally invasive though they differ in that they reduce aqueous production by coagulating ciliary body tissue and are often not included within the MIGS genre.

Endocyclophotocoagulation (ECP) is an *ab interno* cycloablative procedure. An endoscopic camera equipped with an 810 nm diode laser probe in a single 18–20 gauge fibreoptic probe. The ciliary body epithelium is directly visualized during treatment; usually 240–300° of ciliary body are treated with one incision. Two incisions are required for a full 360° treatment [17]. There is no prospective randomized controlled trial on the efficacy of ECP. A case series comparing ECP combined with cataract extraction and cataract extraction alone found slightly lower IOP in the combined group. A retrospective case series comparing ECP with a second glaucoma drainage device (aqueous shunt) in patients with failed previous aqueous shunt surgery found similar IOP outcome at 1 year [18]. Post-operative complications of ECP include inflammation, hypotony, uncontrolled IOP, cystoid macular oedema (10%) and phthisis. Intracameral triamcinolone is suggested to prevent fibrinous inflammation after ECP. Despite its *ab interno* approach, ECP theoretically can cause significant tissue damage and serious complications such as phthisis. Caution should therefore be taken in high-risk eyes.

Micropulse diode laser is a newer method of delivering diode laser to ocular tissue. Conventional laser application is continuous with a single pulse that lasts from 0.1 to 0.5 s. In conventional diode cyclophotocoagulation, the duration of a single laser pulse is usually as long as few seconds. Micropulse mode laser delivers the energy in pulses with pre-set *on* and *off* periods. The *off* period is longer than the *on* period allowing the tissue to cool down and minimize damage. Micropulse laser has been used in the treatment of retinal diseases and glaucoma. In one prospective randomized series, micropulse cyclophotocoagulation is shown to be as efficient, resulting in similar IOP with less complications compared with conventional CPC.

1.5   Overview Summary

Subconjunctival drainage of aqueous humour has been the cornerstone of glaucoma surgery. MIGS devices targeting subconjunctival drainage achieve lower IOP than those targeting Schlemm's canal and suprachoroidal drainage, at the cost of possible bleb-related and higher hypotony-related complications. MIGS targeting the trabecular outflow system such as iStent Trabecular Micro-Bypass Stent or iStent *inject*, Hydrus Microstent and AIT are best suited for patients with moderate OHT or mild to moderate POAG requiring cataract surgery. The IOP-lowering effect of these trabecular devices is limited by episcleral venous pressure (EVP) which limits the maximal IOP reduction to the mid-teens. Subconjunctival draining devices (XEN Gel Implant or PRESERFLO MicroShunt) can be used as solo glaucoma procedure and have better potential to achieve single digit IOP levels. The long-term efficacy of sub-conjunctival MIGS is still unknown as there are few published data on these devices. They both require anti-metabolite (MMC) use as subconjunctival scarring is inevitable with the diversion of aqueous humour to the subconjunctival space. Suprachoroidal drainage devices aim at a potential space where IOP lowering is not limited by EVP and bleb formation is avoided. Scarring in the suprachoroidal space remains an issue. Suprachoroidal devices can potentially be used as an adjunct to traditional glaucoma surgery if further IOP-lowering is required.

References

1. Saheb H, Ahmed II. Micro-invasive glaucoma surgery: current perspectives and future directions. Curr Opin Ophthalmol. 2012;23(2):96–104.
2. Premarket studies of implantable Minimally Invasive Glaucoma Surgical (MIGS) devices: Guidance for Industry and Food and Drug Administration Staff. [cited 2 November 2019]. https://www.fda.gov/media/90950/download.
3. Caprioli J, et al. Special commentary: supporting innovation for safe and effective minimally invasive glaucoma surgery: summary of a joint meeting of the American Glaucoma Society and the Food and Drug Administration, Washington, DC, February 26, 2014. Ophthalmology. 2015;122(9):1795–801.
4. Samuelson TW, et al. Randomized evaluation of the trabecular micro-bypass stent with phacoemulsification in patients with glaucoma and cataract. Ophthalmology. 2011;118(3):459–67.
5. Camras LJ, et al. A novel Schlemm's Canal scaffold increases outflow facility in a human anterior segment perfusion model. Invest Ophthalmol Vis Sci. 2012;53(10):6115–21.
6. Pfeiffer N, et al. A randomized trial of a Schlemm's canal microstent with phacoemulsification for reducing intraocular pressure in open-angle glaucoma. Ophthalmology. 2015;122(7):1283–93.
7. Minckler D, et al. Clinical results with the Trabectome, a novel surgical device for treatment of open-angle glaucoma. Trans Am Ophthalmol Soc. 2006;104:40–50.
8. Grover DS, et al. Gonioscopy-assisted transluminal trabeculotomy, ab interno trabeculotomy: technique report and preliminary results. Ophthalmology. 2014;121(4):855–61.
9. Grover DS, et al. Gonioscopy-assisted transluminal trabeculotomy: an ab interno circumferential trabeculotomy: 24 months follow-up. J Glaucoma. 2018;27(5):393–401.
10. Lewis RA. Ab interno approach to the subconjunctival space using a collagen glaucoma stent. J Cataract Refract Surg. 2014;40(8):1301–6.
11. Batlle JF, et al. Three-year follow-up of a novel aqueous humor MicroShunt. J Glaucoma. 2016;25(2):e58–65.
12. Schlenker MB, et al. Efficacy, safety, and risk factors for failure of standalone ab interno gelatin Microstent implantation versus standalone trabeculectomy. Ophthalmology. 2017;124(11):1579–88.
13. Kerr NM, et al. Ab interno gel implant-associated bleb-related infection. Am J Ophthalmol. 2018;189:96–101.
14. Vold S, et al. Two-year COMPASS trial results: supraciliary microstenting with phacoemulsification in patients with open-angle glaucoma and cataracts. Ophthalmology. 2016;123(10):2103–12.
15. Garcia-Feijoo J, et al. Supraciliary micro-stent implantation for open-angle glaucoma failing topical therapy: 1-year results of a multicenter study. Am J Ophthalmol. 2015;159(6):1075–1081.e1.
16. [cited 2 November 2019]. https://www.alcon.com/cypass-recall-information.
17. Kahook MY, Lathrop KL, Noecker RJ. One-site versus two-site endoscopic cyclophotocoagulation. J Glaucoma. 2007;16(6):527–30.
18. Murakami Y, et al. Endoscopic cyclophotocoagulation versus second glaucoma drainage device after prior aqueous tube shunt surgery. Clin Exp Ophthalmol. 2017;45:241–6.

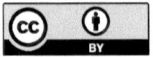

Anatomy of the Aqueous Outflow Drainage Pathways

Kay Lam and Mitchell Lawlor

2.1 Introduction

Minimally invasive glaucoma surgery (MIGS) encompasses a group of procedures aiming to lower intraocular pressure (IOP) with reduced surgical times, more rapid postoperative recovery and a better safety profile compared with traditional filtration surgery. Increasing aqueous humour (AH) outflow may be achieved either through facilitating the existing pathways of Schlemm's canal and the suprachoroidal space or to bypass the normal angle anatomy to create a full thickness fistula into the subconjunctival space. Because of the importance of the anterior chamber angle in the pathogenesis of glaucomatous damage, an understanding of angle anatomy and aqueous outflow structures is critical to surgical planning and device selection for particular glaucoma subtypes. This chapter reviews the clinically relevant anatomy and functionality of the outflow apparatus in the human eye.

2.2 Aqueous Humour Outflow

Intraocular pressure, the main risk factor for glaucoma, is determined by the production, circulation and drainage of AH. The major drainage pathways are the trabecular outflow pathway (conventional outflow) and uveoscleral outflow pathway (unconventional outflow). Aqueous draining through the trabecular outflow system will traverse the trabecular meshwork, through the juxtacanalicular connective tissue, into Schlemm's canal and the collecting channels, and finally into the aqueous veins which then drain into the episcleral venous system. AH draining through the

K. Lam
University of Toronto, Toronto, Ontario, Canada

M. Lawlor (✉)
University of Sydney, Sydney, NSW, Australia
e-mail: mitchell.lawlor@sydney.edu.au

© The Author(s) 2021
C. C. A. Sng, K. Barton (eds.), *Minimally Invasive Glaucoma Surgery*,
https://doi.org/10.1007/978-981-15-5632-6_2

uveoscleral route passes through the ciliary muscle bundles into the suprachoroidal space and then through the sclera into the orbital vessels [1].

The relative contribution of each of these outflow pathways is difficult to determine as it changes depending on the species studied and the method of measurement used. Nonetheless, it is clear that in humans, trabecular meshwork is the major pathway for aqueous outflow accounting for approximately 70–95% of drainage [2, 3]. Uveoscleral outflow in healthy subjects had traditionally been thought to represent a much smaller proportion of AH drainage in healthy humans than primates, though formal aqueous flow studies have reported a value of about 35% in young adults and 3% for individuals over 60 years of age [1, 4]. Aside from the relative contribution of outflow of the two pathways, there are a number of other important differences. Firstly, outflow from the anterior chamber across the trabecular meshwork into Schlemm's canal is pressure dependent, whereas uveoscleral outflow is pressure independent in the physiological range [5, 6]. Secondly, with advancing age, both the trabecular meshwork and uveoscleral outflow facility gradually decline, although there is a relatively greater decline in the uveoscleral contribution to AH drainage overall [2]. To compensate for this, production of AH also decreases with age and therefore IOP is relatively unchanged in the healthy aging human eye [2]. In contrast, eyes with primary open-angle glaucoma have higher outflow resistance in the trabecular outflow pathway than in age-matched normal control eyes, while secretion of AH is not changed [7, 8].

2.3   Trabecular Meshwork

The main ocular structures related to the trabecular outflow pathways are located around the scleral sulcus, a circular groove of the inner sclera, adjacent to the corneoscleral limbus [9]. The sulcus begins at the peripheral termination of Descemet's membrane and extends to the scleral spur, a ridge of inner scleral fibres that run parallel to the limbus, and project inward. This important landmark divides the conventional from the unconventional or uveoscleral outflow. It is best viewed by gonioscopy as no imaging device yet consistently identifies the scleral spur. The scleral spur may also play a role in preventing the ciliary muscle from causing Schlemm's canal to collapse [10]. Schlemm's canal, a circular tube, lies in the outer aspect of the scleral sulcus, while the trabecular meshwork lies at its inner aspect. The trabecular meshwork comprises connective tissue beams or lamellae that are interconnected in several layers to form a porous structure (Fig. 2.1). Each trabecular beam is covered by flat epithelial-like trabecular meshwork cells thought to provide self-cleaning phagocytic activity to maintain the porous structure. Anteriorly, the trabecular beams are attached to the peripheral cornea near the end of Descemet's membrane (Schwalbe's line) and extend posteriorly to ciliary body stroma and scleral spur. The spaces of the trabecular meshwork range in size from 20 to 75 μm and progressively decrease in size posteriorly. The trabecular band covers the internal aspect of Schlemm's canal and is relatively featureless in the unpigmented eye. However, when the meshwork is pigmented, the pigment is concentrated over the canal of Schlemm. Thus, the anterior nonpigmented portion of the trabecular meshwork does not filter, while the posterior pigmented portion of the trabecular meshwork does.

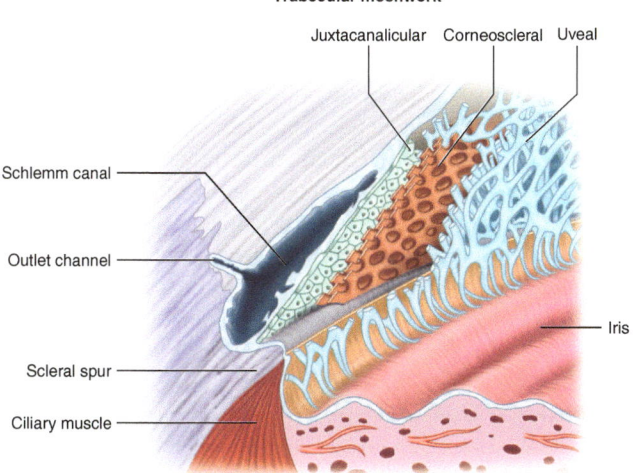

Fig. 2.1 Three layers of trabecular meshwork (shown in cutaway views): uveal, corneoscleral, and juxtacanalicular

This is clinically important as any trans-trabecular devices should target the posterior pigmented trabecular meshwork if the goal is the maximize flow into Schlemm's canal.

2.4   Schlemm's Canal

Schlemm's canal is an endothelial-lined circular tube with one of the highest hydraulic conductivities in the body [6]. Its pores, which range in size from 0.1 to 3 µm in diameter, allow passage not only of AH but also of particulate matter such as cells and ferritin. Additionally, the endothelial lining of Schlemm's canal changes in response to pressure gradient alterations. Elevated IOP leads to an increase in both the number and size of cellular out-pouchings or giant vacuoles while decreased IOP leads to a reduction [11]. AH is transmitted from the trabecular meshwork, through Schlemm's canal, to the distal venous collector system. AH exits Schlemm's canal through collector channels that are spaced at irregular intervals from the outer wall of the canal of Schlemm. They are approximately 25–30 in number and are predominately located in the nasal quadrants [12]. The collector channels ultimately lead to the episcleral venous system; there are two systems of intra-scleral channels: firstly, a direct system of four to six larger veins of Asher that drain directly into the episcleral venous system, and secondly, an indirect system of finer more numerous channels, which form an intrascleral plexus before ultimately draining into the veins of Asher. While the larger conjunctival veins of Asher are readily visible, the intra-scleral plexus is difficult to examine.

Multiple studies suggest that dysfunction of the intrascleral outflow plexus is related to glaucoma; eyes with more advanced disease show downstream collector obstruction or atrophy [13] and functional outflow through human trabecular mesh-work does not occur homogenously—there are regions of preferential flow adjacent to the location of collector channels. Corroborating this are studies showing that the total juxtacanalicular tissue adjacent to collector channels is expanded nearly two-fold compared with the juxtacanalicular regions between collector channels [14]. As canal-based MIGS procedures aim to improve the flow of AH into the venous collec-tor channels, estimating functionality preoperatively or intraoperatively would pro-vide valuable information for both patient selection and prognostication. The finding of an "episcleral venous fluid wave", seen as downstream visible blanching of veins, may be a surrogate marker of anatomic patency of the conventional outflow system from the anterior chamber to the episcleral and conjunctival collectors [15].

2.5   Uveoscleral Outflow

The second route for AH outflow within the eye is through the unconventional out-flow pathway (or uveoscleral pathway). The characterization of this pathway was first provided by Anders Bill in his pioneering work that estimated the outflow using tracer studies [16]. Unlike the trabecular outflow route, the uveoscleral outflow route is not a distinctive structural pathway with channels and tubes. Rather, AH passes through, around and between tissues of the ciliary muscle, supraciliary space and suprachoroidal space. Compared to the conventional pathway, the uveoscleral pathway is less well understood. Nonetheless, new devices that can provide surgical access to these spaces have led to a renewed interest in this anatomical region.

The anterior portion of the ciliary body extends into the chamber angle and there is no epithelial barrier between the anterior chamber and the ciliary muscle [17]. Similarly, there is no continuous cellular layer on the anterior iris face, so aqueous has direct access from the anterior chamber to the interstitial spaces of the ciliary muscle, and then through to the supraciliary and suprachoroidal spaces [16].

The supraciliary space is a narrow area between the outer surface of the ciliary body and the internal surface of the sclera anteriorly. Posteriorly, the suprachoroidal space is located between the choroid and the internal surface of the sclera. This subspace is approximately 30 nm thick and is composed of layers of pigmented col-lagenous processes derived from each tissue, forming a delicate collagen meshwork [18]. This space forms a transitional zone between the choroid and sclera and does not contain overt fluid under normal physiologic conditions.

The mechanism of how fluid from the supraciliary and suprachoroidal spaces exits the eye remains contested: Bill traced the route of radioactive-labelled proteins and other large molecules and proposed that the fluid seeps through sclera and epi-sclera by diffusion into the orbit and then is absorbed by the orbital vasculature [16, 19, 20]. In contrast, Barany and others have suggested that the fluid is osmotically absorbed by the choroid and passes into the vortex veins [21–23].

Evidence of the potential IOP-lowering effect of the suprachoroidal space is derived from the clinical observation that a cyclodialysis cleft from trauma often leads to hypotony. However, harnessing a cyclodialysis cleft to control IOP has remained challenging due to uncontrolled low pressures and then conversely pressure spikes on closure of the cleft. A number of new MIGS devices target this space with the view to obtaining a controlled IOP with appropriate pressure reduction and minimal hypotony.

2.6   Physiological Characteristics of Unconventional Outflow

Aqueous entry into the uveoscleral pathway begins through the interstitial spaces of the ciliary muscle, and ciliary muscle tone has an important influence on outflow. Administration of pilocarpine, which causes contraction of the ciliary muscle fibres and compression of extracellular space, causes uveoscleral outflow to decrease by 90% in cynomolgus monkeys [24]. In contrast, administration of atropine has the opposite effect: it causes relaxation of the muscle fibres, expansion of the extracellular space and thereby increases uveoscleral outflow [25]. Various prostaglandins also increase uveoscleral outflow by modifying the extracellular matrix between ciliary muscle bundles, thus reducing outflow resistance and allowing increased flow through these spaces [26].

Measuring outflow of the uveoscleral pathway is challenging because of intrinsic challenges in measuring the flow rate. Measurements can either be direct or indirect. Direct measurements involve injecting a tracer molecule into the anterior chamber and measuring its accumulation in ocular tissues and blood. While accurate, these tests are invasive and thus not generally suitable for human subjects. Only one study has reported direct measurements of uveoscleral outflow in the living human eye: Bill and Phillips [16] measured outflow in two normal eyes that were not receiving topical pilocarpine or atropine and found uveoscleral outflow accounted for 4–14% of total outflow.

Indirect techniques calculate uveoscleral outflow using a modified Goldmann equation, which requires the measurement of four other parameters, each with inherent variability. This method tends to yield large standard deviations with considerable variability.

These limitations notwithstanding, the uveoscleral outflow pathway appears to be relatively insensitive to IOP differences, even over the range of 4 to 35 mmHg [19]. This observation in part has meant that the majority of surgical targets to lower IOP have focused on the pressure-dependent trabecular outflow system. However, once the ciliary muscle is bypassed (through a shunt or a cyclodialysis cleft), most of the resistance it offers is lost [27] and the uveoscleral pathway becomes pressure dependent, with outflow increasing fourfold [28]. When the uveoscleral pathway is turned into a pressure-dependent pathway, as noted above, its capability of lowering IOP is so significant that the postoperative IOP can reach the low teens or single digits [29–31].

2.7   Conjunctival Lymphatic System

The human lymphatic system plays an important role in body fluid homeostasis, lipid absorption and immune function [31–33]. Fundamentally, the lymphatic system removes excess arterial fluid that is unable to be absorbed by the venous system from the interstitial space and acts to enhance immune surveillance. Traditionally seen as passive channels for fluid and immune cells, recent discoveries have drastically changed our view of lymphatic vasculature, which lags far behind our knowledge of the vascular system. Lymphatic vessels are now appearing to have diverse functions with remarkable specialization depending on tissue microenvironment [34].

Despite this limited knowledge, it appears conjunctival lymphatics are particularly important for the success of glaucoma surgical outcomes [35–37]. In the normal eye, conjunctival lymphatics are not involved in AH flow pathways, and lymphatics have no communication with conjunctival veins [38]. However, glaucoma filtering surgery alters the normal pathways. Aqueous humour is diverted into the subconjunctival space, which is equivalent to interstitial tissue fluid, where conjunctival lymphatic vessels exist. Animal studies confirm that the presence of lymphatic drainage pathways is associated with persistence of subconjunctival drainage pathways, which in turn play a key role in determining surgical outcomes of glaucoma filtration surgery [39]. Thus, understanding conjunctival lymphatic drainage is critical to optimize glaucoma therapeutic interventions.

Conjunctival lymphatics remain difficult to study because of their transparent, colourless nature and very thin vessel walls with absent basement membrane or pericytes. The lymphatic system is a series of unidirectional, thin-walled vessels that transport lymph to the lymphatic nodes, which eventually empty into the blood veins via the thoracic duct.

Conjunctival lymphatics in monkeys start with blind-ended terminals located in the superficial conjunctiva between the epithelium and Tenon's capsule [40]. These tubular vessels are of uneven calibre with numerous branch communications that are responsible for the initial drainage of interstitial fluid. The mechanism of fluid uptake appears to be transient fluid pressure gradients between the interstitial fluid and the initial lymphatic [41, 42]. The fluid then drains into valved precollectors, which are mostly located in the deep layer under Tenon's capsule. These connect to larger collectors and eventually empty into the preauricular and submaxillary lymph nodes [43, 44]. The lymphatics appear to be relatively evenly distributed in the bulbar conjunctiva, with no difference between each quadrant or between the limbus or fornix regions.

Our knowledge of conjunctival lymphatics is still rudimentary, but an understanding of this system's role in interstitial fluid drainage is crucial to optimizing and targeting aqueous drainage in glaucoma therapy. Understanding the lymphatic vessels structure and function, distribution in the conjunctiva and eventually their functional assessment prior to filtration surgery will have significant implications for surgical glaucoma treatments that create a conjunctival bleb.

2.8   Conclusions

Lowering IOP has been central to glaucoma care for over a century. New surgical devices are able to exploit different aspects of aqueous outflow to reduce IOP. A complete understanding of outflow pathways is important to develop new treatment strategies, improve current ones, and to better target the right operation for particular glaucoma subtypes.

References

1. Alm A, Nilsson SF. Uveoscleral outflow—a review. Exp Eye Res. 2009;88(4):760–8.
2. Toris CB, Koepsell SA, Yablonski ME, et al. Aqueous humor dynamics in ocular hyptertensive patients. J Glaucoma. 2002;11(3):253.
3. Toris CB, Yablonski ME, Wang YL, et al. Aqueous humor dynamics in the aging human eye. Am J Ophthalmol. 1999;127(4):407.
4. Townsend DJ, Brubaker RF. Immediate effect of epinephrine on aqueous formation in the normal human eye as measured by fluorophotometry. Invest Ophthalmol Vis Sci. 1980;19(3):256.
5. Brubaker RF. Measurement of uveoscleral outflow in humans. J Glaucoma. 2001;10(5 Suppl 1):S45.
6. Johnson M. What controls aqueous humour outflow resistance? Exp Eye Res. 2006;82:545.
7. Brubaker RF. Flow of aqueous humor in humans. Invest Ophthalmol Vis Sci. 1991;32:3145.
8. Larsson LI, Rettig ES, Sheridan PT, et al. Aqueous humor dynamics in low-tension glaucoma. Am J Ophthalmol. 1993;116:590.
9. Tamm ER. The trabecular meshwork outflow pathways: structural and functional aspects. Exp Eye Res. 2009;88:648.
10. Moses RA, Grodski WJ Jr. The scleral spur and scleral roll. Invest Ophthalmol Vis Sci. 1977;16(10):925.
11. Johnstone MA, Grant WG. Pressure-dependent changes in structures of the aqueous outflow system of human and monkey eyes. Am J Ophthalmol. 1973;75(3):365–83.
12. Kagemann L, Wollstein G, Ishikawa H, et al. Identification and assessment of Schlemm's canal by spectral-domain optical coherence tomography. Invest Ophthalmol Vis Sci. 2010;51:4054–9.
13. Nesterov AP. Pathological physiology of primary open angle glaucoma: the aqueous circulation. In: Cairns JE, editor. Glaucoma, vol. I. New York: Grune and Stratton; 1986. p. 335–6.
14. Hann CR, Fautsch MP. Preferential fluid flow in the human trabecular meshwork near collector channels. Invest Ophthalmol Vis Sci. 2009;50(4):1692–7.
15. Fellman RL, Feuer WJ, Grover DS. Episcleral venous fluid wave correlates with trabectome outcomes: intraoperative evaluation of the trabecular outflow pathway. Ophthalmology. 2015;122:2385–91.e1.
16. Bill A, Phillips CI. Uveoscleral drainage of aqueous humour in human eyes. Exp Eye Res. 1971;12:275–81.
17. Nilsson SFE. The uveoscleral outflow routes. Eye. 1997;11:149–54.
18. Hogan MH, Alvarado JA, Weddell JE. Histology of the human eye—an atlas and textbook. Philadelphia: Saunders; 1971. p. 320.
19. Bill A. Conventional and uveo-scleral drainage of aqueous humour in the cynomolgus monkey (*Macaca irus*) at normal and high intraocular pressures. Exp Eye Res. 1966;5:45–54.
20. Bill A. Blood circulation and fluid dynamics in the eye. Physiol Rev. 1975;55:383–416.
21. Barany EH. Pseudofacility and uveoscleral outflow routes. Munich: Basel, Karger; 1967.

22. Pederson JE, Gassterland DE, MacLellan HM. Uveoscleral aqueous outflow in the rhesus monkey: importance of uveal reabsorption. Invest Ophthalmol Vis Sci. 1977;16:1008–17.
23. Sherman SH, Green K, Laties AM. The fate of anterior chamber fluorescein in the monkey eye. 1. The anterior chamber outflow pathways. Exp Eye Res. 1978;27:159–73.
24. Crawford K, Kaufman PL. Pilocarpine antagonizes prostaglandin F2 alpha-induced ocular hypotension in monkeys. Evidence for enhancement of uveoscleral outflow by prostaglandin F2 alpha. Arch Ophthalmol. 1987;105(8):1112–6.
25. Bill A, Walinder P. The effects of pilocarpine on the dynamics of aqueous humor in a primate (Macaca irus). Investig Ophthalmol. 1966;5(2):170–5.
26. Lutgen-Drecoll E, Tamm E. Morphological study of the anterior segment of cynomolgus monkey eyes following treatment with prostaglandin F2a. Exp Eye Res. 1988;47(5):761–9.
27. Bill A. The routes for bulk drainage of aqueous humor in rabbits with and without cyclodialysis. Doc Ophthalmol. 1966;20:157–69.
28. Suguro K, Toris CB, Pederson JE. Uveoscleral outflow following cyclodialysis cleft in the monkey eye using a fluorescent tracer. Invest Ophthalmol Vis Sci. 1985;26:810–3.
29. Emi K, Pederson JE, Toris CB. Hydrostatic pressure of the suprachoroidal space. Invest Ophthalmol Vis Sci. 1989;30:233–8.
30. Skaat A, Sagiv O, Kinori M, Simon GJ, Goldenfeld M, Melamed S. Gold Micro-Shunt implants versus Ahmed Glaucoma Valve: long-term outcomes of a prospective randomized clinical trial. J Glaucoma. 2016;2:155–61.
31. Gausas RE, Gonnering RS, Lemke BN, et al. Identification of human orbital lymphatics. Ophthal Plast Reconstr Surg. 1999;15:252–9.
32. Schmid-Schonbein GW. Microlymphatics and lymph flow. Physiol Rev. 1990;70(4):987–1028.
33. Steenbergen JM, Lash JM, Bohlen HG. Role of a lymphatic system in glucose absorption and the accompanying microvascular hyperemia. Am J Phys. 1994;267(4 Pt 1):G529–35.
34. Petrova TV, Koh GY. Organ-specific lymphatic vasculature: from development to pathophysiology. J Exp Med. 2018;215(1):35–49.
35. Ritch R, Shields MB, Krupin T. The glaucomas. St Louis: The C.V. Mosby Company; 1989. p. 1–748.
36. Teng CC, Chi HH, Katzin HM. Histology and mechanism of filtering operations. Am J Ophthalmol. 1959;47:16–34.
37. Singh D. A new clue to lymphatic drainage. Rev Ophthalmol. 2002;9:12.
38. Yu D-Y, Morgan WH, Sun X, et al. The critical role of the conjunctiva in glaucoma filtration surgery. Prog Retin Eye Res. 2009;28:303–28.
39. Morgan WH, Balaratnasingam C, Guibilato A, et al. The use of trypan blue as a tracer to outline aqueous flow. J Ophthalmol Photogr. 2005;27:79–81.
40. Guo W, Zhu Y, Yu PK, et al. Quantitative study of the topographic distribution of conjunctival lymphatic vessels in the monkey. Exp Eye Res. 2012;94:90–7.
41. Moriondo A, Mukenge AS, Negrini D. Transmural pressure in rate initial subpleural lymphatics during spontaneous or mechanical ventilation. Am J Physiol Heart Circ Physiol. 2005;289:H269.
42. Negrin D, Moriondo A, Mukenge S. Transmural pressure during cardiogenic oscillations in rodent diaphragmatic lymphatic vessels. Lymph Res Biol. 2004;2:69–81.
43. Singh D, Singh RSJ, Singh K, et al. The conjunctival lymphatics system. Ann Ophthalmol. 2003;35:99–104.
44. Sugar HS, Riazi A, Schaffner R. The bulbar conjunctival lymphatics and their clinical significance. Trans Am Acad Ophthalmol Otolaryngol. 1957;61:212–23.

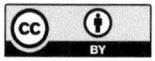

iStent: Trabecular Micro-Bypass Stent

3

Christine L. Larsen and Thomas W. Samuelson

3.1 Device Design

The iStent (or iStent Trabecular Micro-Bypass Stent) (Glaukos Corporation, San Clemente, USA) has become a popular device within the realm of minimally invasive glaucoma surgery (MIGS). These procedures are known to have a higher safety profile and a more rapid recovery time in comparison to more invasive filtering surgery. MIGS procedures have demonstrated the ability to both reduce IOP and a patient's need for medications, a significant benefit considering concerns regarding compliance rates among glaucoma patients [1]. Unlike many other surgical interventions for glaucoma, iStent implantation does not diminish the superlative visual and refractive outcomes inherent to modern phacoemulsification. As with many MIGS procedures, stent placement is minimally traumatic to the target tissue and spares the conjunctiva via an *ab interno* approach.

The iStent was developed by Glaukos (Glaukos Corporation, San Clemente, CA, USA) with the first implantation in the United States performed in 2005 [2]. The stent is designed to fit into and remain within Schlemm's canal. Made from non-ferromagnetic titanium, it consists of an inlet (or "snorkel") connected at a 40° angle to the implanted portion. The stent itself is then attached to the tip of a 26-gauge disposable insertion instrument, which has been sterilized by gamma radiation (Fig. 3.1a, b). The inserter tubing contains four-finger extensions which grasp the stent. A pointed end of the device facilitates entry into the canal and the direction of this point corresponds to the designation of a right or left-handed model (GTS100R and GTS100L, respectively). Depending on the preference of the surgeon, both "right" and "left" iStents have been developed to ease implantation. The segment residing within the canal includes a half cylinder opening, which combined with heparin coating, helps to prevent blockage or fibrosis. Three retention arches

C. L. Larsen (✉) · T. W. Samuelson
Minnesota Eye Consultants, P.A., Bloomington, MN, USA
e-mail: cllarsen@mneye.com

© The Author(s) 2021
C. C. A. Sng, K. Barton (eds.), *Minimally Invasive Glaucoma Surgery*,
https://doi.org/10.1007/978-981-15-5632-6_3

Fig. 3.1 The direction of the pointed end with the inserter held upright (button on the top) designates right or left-handed models. (Copyright Glaukos Corporation, San Clemente, CA, USA; reproduced with permission)

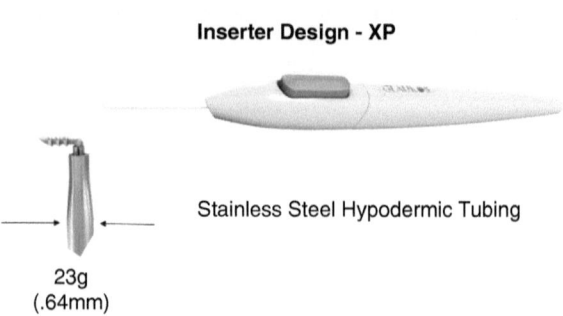

Fig. 3.2 Implanted in the trabecular meshwork, the stent allows aqueous humor to flow into Schlemm's canal. (Copyright Glaukos Corporation, San Clemente, CA, USA; reproduced with permission)

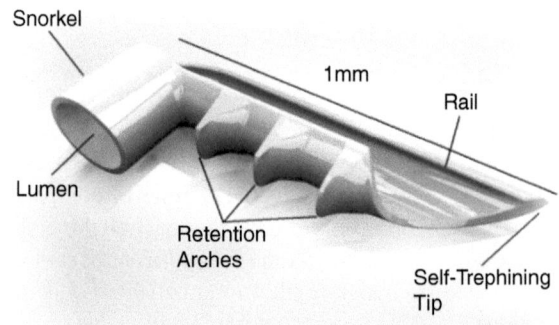

help to ensure that the device will be held in place within the canal. The implant is 1.0 mm in length, 0.33 mm in height, and with a weight of 60 µg. The snorkel has a length of 0.25 mm and bore diameter of 120 µm [3] (Fig. 3.2).

The iStent *inject* system (Glaukos Corporation, San Clemente, CA, USA), a second-generation device or G2, consists of an apical head connected to a narrow thorax that is attached to a wider flange. Currently, the smallest medical implant approved for use in the human body, the implant is 360 µm in length and with a diameter of 230 µm (Fig. 3.3a, b). The central inlet and outlet lumen has a diameter of 80 µm. The head is inserted directly into the canal without the necessity to adjust the angle for implantation. It resides within the canal and contains four inlets for fluid passage, each with a diameter of 50 µm. The 23-gauge stainless steel injector contains two stents for implantation in the nasal angle, at a distance of approximately 30–60° (Fig. 3.4). The iStent *inject* was approved for use in Europe in 2006, and FDA approval in the United States was obtained in June 2018.

The iStent works at the level of the trabecular meshwork (TM). Research regarding the physiology of primary open-angle glaucoma (POAG) has demonstrated that the diseased juxtacanalicular meshwork is the primary site of reduced outflow facility resulting from increased outflow resistance [4]. Implantation of the device allows

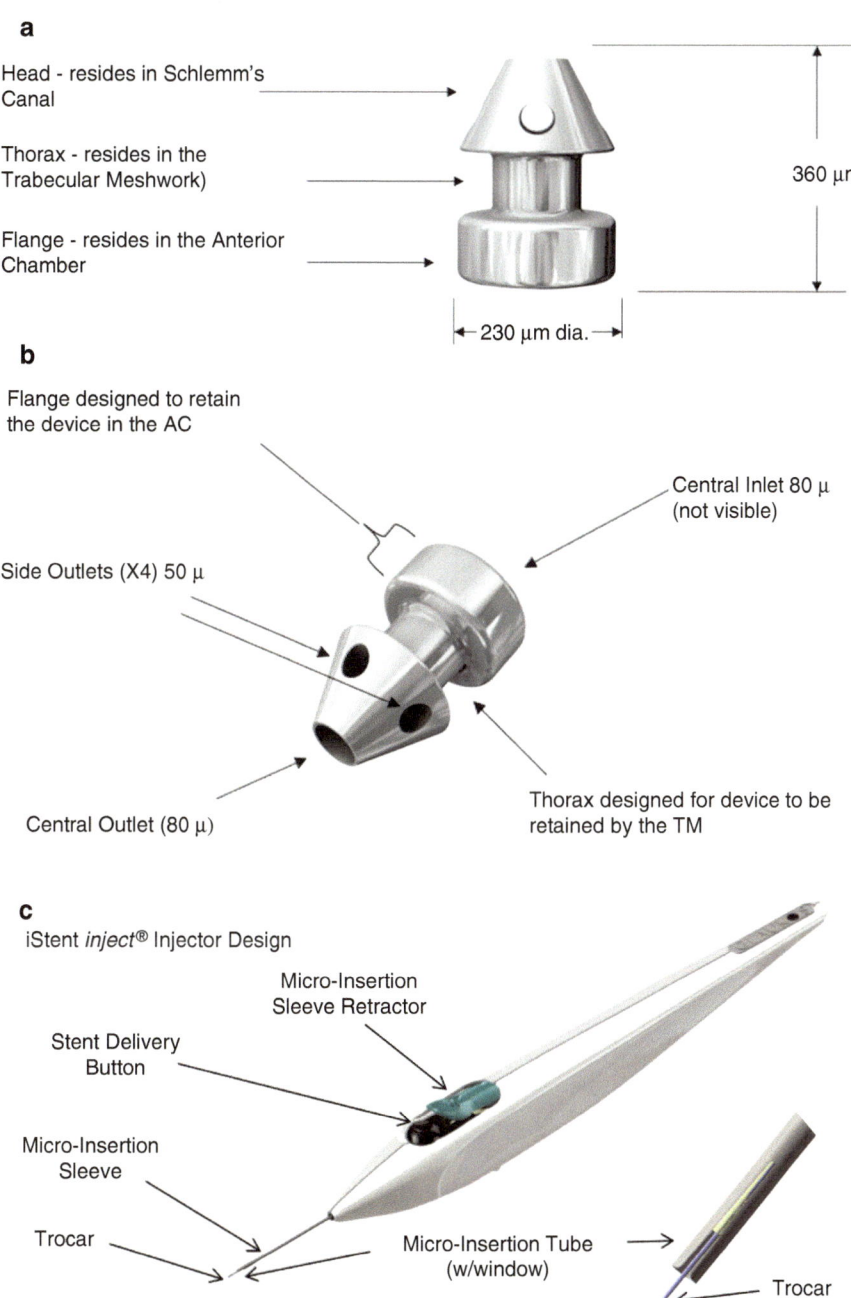

a

Head - resides in Schlemm's Canal

Thorax - resides in the Trabecular Meshwork)

Flange - resides in the Anterior Chamber

360 μm

←— 230 μm dia. —→

b

Flange designed to retain the device in the AC

Central Inlet 80 μ (not visible)

Side Outlets (X4) 50 μ

Central Outlet (80 μ)

Thorax designed for device to be retained by the TM

c

iStent *inject*® Injector Design

Micro-Insertion Sleeve Retractor

Stent Delivery Button

Micro-Insertion Sleeve

Trocar

Micro-Insertion Tube (w/window)

Trocar

Fig. 3.3 (**a, b**) The iStent *inject* is the smallest known medical implant used in the human body. (**c**) The trochar of the injector system pierces the trabecular meshwork, allowing the distal portion of the stent to be injected into Schlemm's canal. (Copyright Glaukos Corporation, San Clemente, CA, USA; reproduced with permission)

Fig. 3.4 The iStent *inject* system allows for implantation of two preloaded trabecular micro-bypass stents with a single entry. (Copyright Thomas Samuelson, MD; reproduced with permission)

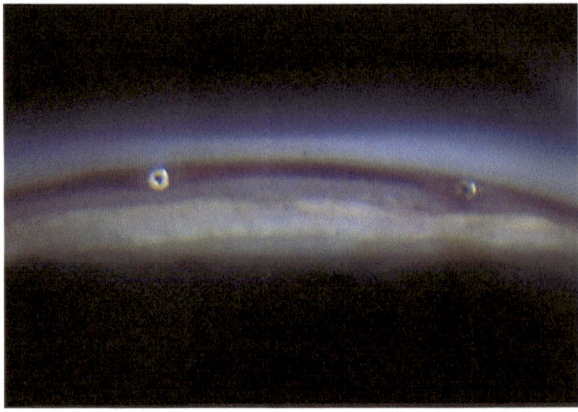

for aqueous to bypass the increased TM resistance to outflow and provides a direct pathway into Schlemm's canal and the subsequent collector channels. The postoperative IOP would not be expected to fall below the episcleral venous pressure (EVP), which has been reported in different studies to range between 7.6 and 9.1 mmHg [5–7] and may be elevated in some glaucoma patients [8]. This is a limitation in the treatment of patients with very low target IOP; however, a benefit in the avoidance of hypotonous sequelae.

Zhou et al. demonstrated the effectiveness of trabecular bypass on outflow facility and IOP [9]. A series of equations explored this relationship and demonstrated that in normal healthy eyes, the outflow facility increases by 13 and 26% in the presence of a unidirectional and bidirectional bypass, respectively. The IOP could be reduced to physiologic levels with outflow facility enhancement. Bahler et al. looked at the effect of a trabecular meshwork bypass on IOP in cultured human anterior segments [10]. A single stent placed into Schlemm's canal provided the greatest change in pressure (21.4 ± 3.8 mmHg to 12.4 ± 4.2, $P < 0.001$) with the addition of more stents providing further lowering of pressure, but to a lesser degree.

Similarly, Bahler et al. also addressed the influences of the iStent *inject* on the outflow facility of cultured human anterior segments [11]. Outflow facility was shown to increase and IOP to decrease with a single stent placement. An additional increase in outflow facility was demonstrated with the placement of a second stent.

3.2   Patient Selection

In 2012, the FDA approved the iStent for use in combination with cataract extraction for patients with mild-to-moderate open-angle glaucoma who were using between 1 and 3 ocular hypotensive medications. The stent is currently approved in Europe as a stand-alone procedure or for use in combined cataract/MIGS procedures.

Ideal candidates are those with stable and well-controlled or modestly uncontrolled disease. Patients demonstrating rapid progression or extreme elevation of IOP on their current medication regimen may require more aggressive surgical intervention such as filtration surgery. Optimal patients typically need pressure lowering, but not to an extreme level. In addition to improving IOP, another goal is to reduce the dependency on topical medication, but not necessarily advance the aggressiveness of treatment.

Patients with a very shallow anterior chamber with peripheral anterior synechiae are typically avoided, as implantation requires access to Schlemm's Canal. Although the angle will be deeper once the native lens has been removed, implantation in shallow anterior chambers can be more difficult with an increased risk of iris or endothelial damage. Secondary glaucomas related to elevated episcleral venous pressure are less ideal, as successful outcomes require an otherwise functional outflow system. Patients with neovascular glaucoma are contraindicated because of both the increased bleeding risk and reduced function of the outflow system [12].

As the surgeon is first developing their implantation skills and becoming more comfortable with the procedure, it may be of benefit to select patients who would do well with cataract surgery alone. These patients will still likely do well postoperatively should implantation be unsuccessful. Other favorable traits for initial cases might include highly cooperative individuals with at least moderate pigmentation of the TM and easily identifiable angle structures. If a surgeon favors right or left eyes for phacoemulsification, he or she is likely to favor such eyes for initial iStent cases as well.

3.3   Surgical Technique

Proficiency with intraoperative gonioscopy is imperative to success with iStent implantation. For surgeons who do not perform gonioscopy often, it is useful to examine patients in clinic to better familiarize oneself with the angle anatomy. Practicing intraoperative gonioscopy during routine cataract cases can also be of benefit prior to implanting the first stent. Gently touching the anterior meshwork with a viscoelastic cannula can help one become more comfortable with the hand positioning.

Upon completion of cataract surgery and implantation of the IOL, injection of a miotic helps to pull the iris away from the angle and insertion of viscoelastic material will aid in maintaining the anterior chamber. For initial cases, it is desirable to remove all viscoelastic from the retropupillary space and capsular bag before the pupil is constricted. Once more experience is achieved, many surgeons will choose to wait until the iStent has been successfully implanted before the viscoelastic is removed and the miotic instilled. The patient's head and the operating microscope are rotated 30–40° in opposite directions to facilitate a gonioscopic view of the angle. The surgical gonioprism is placed on the cornea with a coupling solution (goniosol, viscoelastic) and the angle is viewed under high magnification. Care to avoid pressure on the eye with the goniolens is important, as resultant corneal striae will impede the view. Likewise, the surgeon should not place pressure on the wound with the insertion trochar to avoid expressing viscoelastic from the eye. Once a clear view of the trabecular meshwork is achieved, the applicator is inserted into the anterior chamber through the clear corneal incision and advanced across the anterior chamber toward the nasal angle. As mentioned previously, there are two different designs designating the direction of the pointed end. The intent of the unique iStent design is that after implantation, the body of the stent points toward the inferior angle such that right stents are used in right eyes and left stents are used in left eyes (Fig. 3.5). Evidence that right or left orientation makes any clinical difference, however, is lacking. As such, most surgeons believe that right- and left-hand models are interchangeable (i.e., right and left iStents can be used in both right and left eyes) depending on what feels more comfortable (forehand or backhand) in the dominant hand of the surgeon.

The anterior 1/3 of the trabecular meshwork is approached at a 15° angle and is perforated by the tip and advanced into the canal. By slightly adjusting the angle after perforation (lowering the heel and raising the toe), the stent will slide into the canal more easily. A "landing strip" technique has recently been described to help guide implantation. Zheng et al. suggested using a 25-guage microvitreoretinal blade to bisect the trabecular meshwork for less than 1 clock hour, thus creating a guide for assistance stent placement [13]. Once securely positioned with the ridges of stent covered by meshwork tissue, the device is released by pushing the button on the applicator. Subtle posterior pressure and relaxing of the hand will ensure a stable release.

After release, the iStent should appear to be well seated within the canal. The device will be viewed running parallel to the iris plane (Fig. 3.6a, b). The applicator tip is used to gently push the inlet to verify it has memory (i.e., with minimal displacement, it will return to the original position). After successful placement, viscoelastic material should be thoroughly removed at the conclusion of the case.

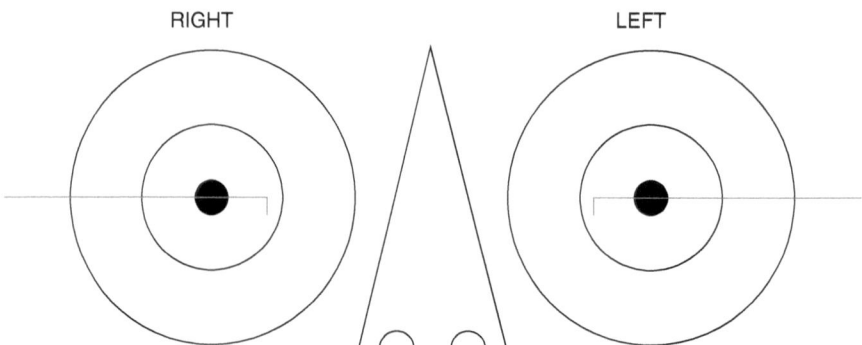

Fig. 3.5 The intent of the unique iStent design is that after implantation, the body of the stent points toward the inferior angle such that right stents are used in right eyes and left stents are used in the left eyes. Evidence that right or left orientation makes any clinical difference is lacking and most surgeons now believe that right- and left-hand models are interchangeable. (Copyright Glaukos Corporation, San Clemente, CA, USA; reproduced with permission)

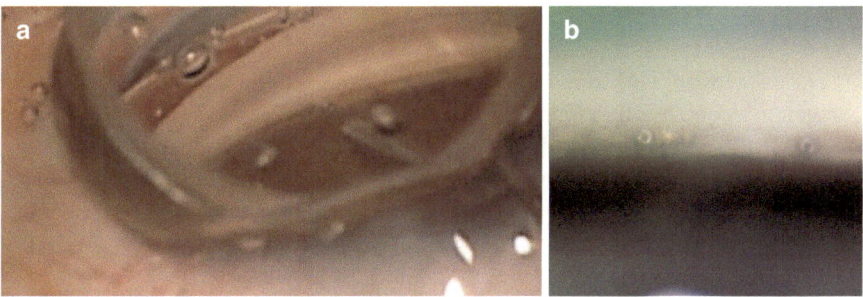

Fig. 3.6 (**a**) With successful implantion, the iStent is viewed running parallel to the iris plane with retention arches covered by trabecular meshwork tissue (Copyright Thomas Samuelson, MD; reproduced with permission). (**b**) Gonioscopy photograph of two iStents showing superficial placement of the left stent as evidenced by visible retention arches. The right stent is well placed in Schlemm's canal and the retention arches are obscured by the pigmented trabecular meshwork. (Copyright Chelvin Sng, FRCSEd; reproduced with permission)

3.3.1 Avoiding Complications and Surgical Pearls

Advantages of the iStent procedure include sparing of the conjunctiva and avoidance of the long-term complications and short-term risks associated with trabeculectomy and tube shunt surgery. More specifically, issues of hypotony are avoided because episcleral backpressure remains.

With any surgical procedure, however, adverse events can occur. The larger studies involving the iStent have not demonstrated any significant added risk in comparison to cataract surgery alone. Publications from the iStent Study User Group at both 12 and 24 months showed the overall incidence of adverse events and long-term safety profile was similar between cataract surgery alone and cataract surgery with iStent implantation. Unanticipated adverse device effects were not seen [14, 15].

Now with several years of use and data, there have been a few case reports published describing isolated complications. Sandhu et al. reported the first documented case of delayed-onset and recurrent hyphema after iStent placement [16]. Two episodes of spontaneous hyphema were seen within a 19-month postoperative period. There were no associations with anticoagulants, stent malposition, or angle abnormalities, and the episodes were thought to be related to ocular pressure from sleeping position that was reduced upon waking. Regarding implantation, Mantravadi et al. reported a case of inadvertent implantation of an iStent into the supracilliary space [17]. An iridodialysis cleft was created at the time of attempted stent repositioning. The stent was no longer visible intraoperatively and was subsequently identified in the supracilliary space via ultrasound biomicroscopy. No adverse sequelae were identified related to the malposition.

Although the overall risks and adverse events seen postoperatively with iStent placement are similar to cataract surgery alone, there are some intraoperative complexities that may be encountered and steps that can be taken to ensure a successful implantation.

When viewing the angle gonioscopically at the time of stent placement, Schlemm's canal is often highlighted by blood within. This is a benefit in regard to canal identification, but can also impede the view as blood is released after perforation of the trabecular meshwork. If the angle anatomy becomes obscured, irrigation and aspiration may be utilized to clear the blood or additional viscoelastic may push it out of the way. Blood visualized flowing out of the snorkel after insertion is a good but somewhat inconsistent sign, indicating correct positioning within the canal (Fig. 3.7) Quite often blood reflux is not seen until after viscoelastic removal prior to re-pressurization of the eye. Similarly, transient blanching of the episcleral vessels has been proposed as means to confirm accurate stent placement and may be a prognostic indicator (Fig. 3.8a, b). Fellman et al. first described this phenomenon in patients undergoing combined phacoemulsification–trabectome surgery and believed the episcleral venous fluid wave signifies intraoperative structural patency of the conventional outflow system [18]. They were subsequently able to demonstrate a diffuse venous wave resulted in lower IOP, fewer glaucoma

Fig. 3.7 Blood visualized exiting the snorkel of the device can be an indicator of accurate placement. (Copyright Thomas Samuelson, MD; reproduced with permission)

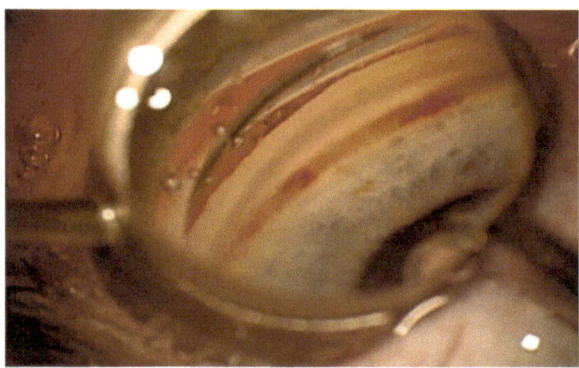

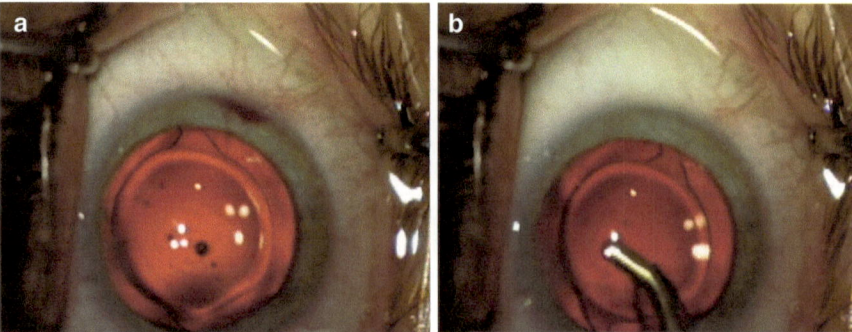

Fig. 3.8 (**a, b**) Episcleral vasculature before and after successful iStent placement. The episcleral venous wave demonstrates a structurally intact collector channel system. (Copyright Christine Larsen, MD; reproduced with permission)

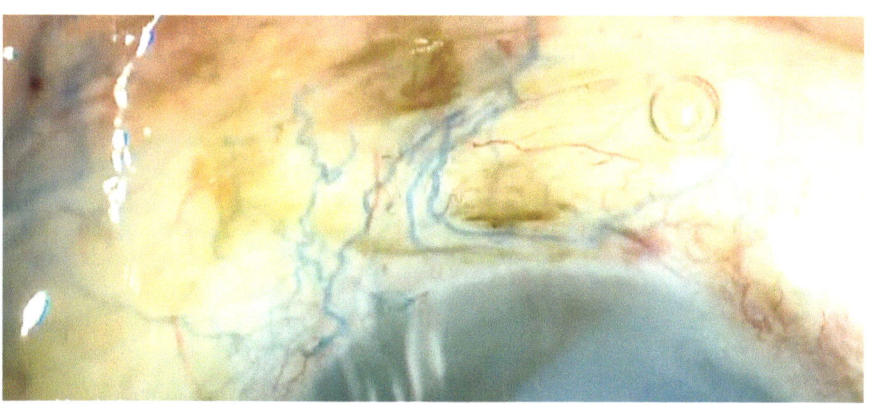

Fig. 3.9 Injection of trypan blue dye in the anterior chamber clearly delineates the aqueous veins in an eye with two well-placed iStent Trabecular Micro-Bypass Stents. (Copyright Chelvin Sng, FRCSEd; reproduced with permission)

medications, and lower requirement for additional surgery in 68 eyes of a similar patient population [19]. Similarly, trypan blue dye (Vision Blue, DORC International) can be used to confirm correct stent placement by allowing the delineation of aqueous veins in blue (Fig. 3.9). This finding has led to the idea of targeted placement. Identification of larger episcleral veins at the beginning of surgery may allow the surgeon to preferentially position the iStent at this location. The same idea is employed under gonioscopic view of the angle. Areas of increased pigmentation or blood within the canal may signify proximity to a collector channel [20] and would thus be an ideal target for iStent placement. Unfortunately, no method exists to evaluate the patency and capacity of collector channels before deciding to proceed with canal surgery. There is also no current mechanism to modulate wound healing in the canal, which can be a detriment to the surgical success of MIGS procedures. The second-generation device, iStent *inject* obviates the need for intelligent placement to some extent by virtue of the fact that more than one stent is placed increasing the likelihood of reaching collector channels.

As discussed earlier, avoidance of patients with shallow anterior chambers can help prevent issues with endothelial damage or iris root tears. Should these occur, the stent can still be safely inserted, however, the patient may require more intensive postoperative care should transient corneal edema or hyphema result.

Another important precaution relates to the re-grasping maneuver should the iStent need repositioning. While the stent can be readily re-grasped by the inserter, care must be exercised to be certain that the re-grasping prongs do not accidentally grasp the iris along with the stent. Should this occur, an iridodialysis or iris trauma could result.

After intraocular lens placement, viscoelastic should be completely removed from both the anterior chamber and posterior to the iris and IOL. Successful evacuation of all viscoelastic is the most important final step in preventing early postoperative IOP spikes. After the instillation of a miotic, the amount of viscoelastic reintroduced into the anterior chamber should be enough to provide stability and adequate visualization of the canal without resulting in pressure on the meshwork. After stent placement, the viscoelastic is again thoroughly removed. Some surgeons may elect to place the iStent prior to phacoemulsification. One advantage of this strategy is that viscoelastic management subsequently proceeds as per usual for standard cataract surgery. In addition, the view through the cornea may be clearer prior to cataract removal.

3.3.2 Postoperative Management

Open-angle glaucoma patients are more susceptible to intraocular pressure elevation after surgery regardless of whether cataract surgery is performed alone or in combination with iStent placement. In addition to an early postoperative pressure increase related to retained viscoelastic, these patients are also at increased risk of experiencing a steroid response. It may be beneficial to taper steroids more rapidly. The supplemental benefit of a nonsteroidal anti-inflammatory agent often allows earlier discontinuation of steroidal agents.

It will typically take about 6–8 weeks from the surgery date to reach a new steady state for intraocular pressure. Glaucoma medications may be discontinued on a case-by-case basis. Lower risk eyes and those with a lower medication burden (i.e., 1–2 topical medications) may be able to have all glaucoma treatment withdrawn. For those requiring two or more medications or a higher risk patient, medications should be discontinued more cautiously and in a stepwise fashion.

Other potentially encountered issues in the postoperative period include the presence of a hyphema, with possible occlusion of the stent with blood, or occlusion by iris tissue (Fig. 3.10). Treatment of a hyphema in this case is no different than the normal standard of care. Should the stent become blocked with iris tissue, neodymium:YAG laser or argon laser can be utilized to successfully clear the blockage should IOP become uncontrolled [14, 21].

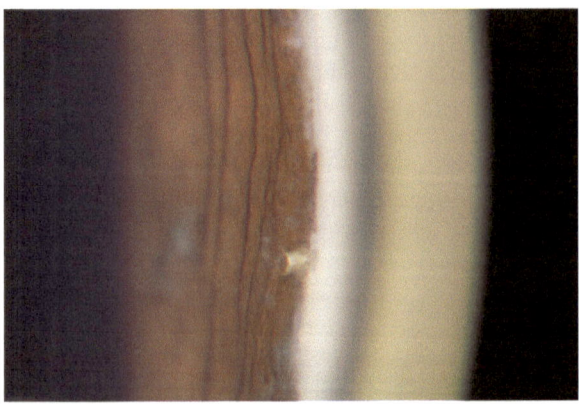

Fig. 3.10 Gonioscopy photograph showing complete iStent occlusion with iris in an eye with angle-closure disease. (Copyright Chelvin Sng, FRCSEd; reproduced with permission)

3.4   Safety, Efficacy, and Clinical Results

3.4.1   iStent Trabecular Micro-Bypass Stent

The US iStent Study Group performed a large comparative study in POAG patients already undergoing planned cataract surgery to compare the effect between cataract removal alone and cataract removal in combination with iStent placement [14]. Prior to this study, several pilot studies had been performed demonstrating the effectiveness of iStent implantation at lowering IOP.

The initial results of the iStent Study Group, the largest study to date, were published in 2011 [14]. The study involved 239 patients with 116 patients receiving the stent. Patients involved in the study were those with mild–moderate glaucoma who had an unmedicated IOP between 22 and 36 mmHg. The primary efficacy measure was defined as unmedicated IOP ≤ 21 mmHg at 1 year and was seen in 72% of treatment eyes versus 50% of controls. A secondary outcome was unmedicated IOP reduction $\geq 20\%$ at 1 year and was seen in 66% of treatment eyes versus 48% of controls. Approximately half as many patients in the iStent group were using topical drops compared to the cataract only group at 1 year, suggesting that the iStent may delay or eliminate the need for drops after cataract surgery (a mean reduction in medications of 1.4 for iStent group and 1.0 for cataract only group).

The incidence of adverse events seen with cataract surgery plus iStent placement versus cataract surgery alone was similar in the iStent Study Group. No unanticipated adverse device effects were seen. The goal of improved vision was achieved in $\geq 95\%$ of subjects for both groups.

A subsequent paper published by the iStent Study Group looked at the same end points at 24 months [15]. It found that the proportion of patients with an IOP of <21 mmHg without medication was significantly higher in the stent group. The mean IOP was stable between the 1 and 2 year end points in the stent group, however, was slightly increased in the control group (17.0 ± 3.1 vs. 17.8 ± 3.3). The total number of hypotensive medications was shown to be significantly less in the stent group at 12 months. This finding was additionally maintained at 24 months, however, was no longer statistically significant. It should be noted that the original study was only powered to detect a difference out to 1 year. Again, postoperative complications and adverse events were similar between groups at 24 months (Table 3.1).

Several publications have since demonstrated similar findings in terms of iStent efficacy and safety profile [22–24]. A summary of the randomized controlled trials and case series to date is provided in Table 3.2. The most common complication across all studies was stent obstruction or malposition, which in general did not result in any adverse sequelae.

3.4.2   iStent *inject*

Fea et al. conducted a randomized, prospective, multicenter evaluation which suggested that treatment with two iStent *inject* devices is comparable to medical

Table 3.1 Postoperative ocular complications reported in the iStent User Group at 24 months

Complication	iStent group (n = 116)	Control group (n = 117)
Anticipated early postoperative event[a]	20 (17.2%)	22 (18.8%)
Posterior capsule opacification	7 (6%)	12 (10.3%)
Elevated IOP	4 (3.4%)	5 (4.3%)
Elevated IOP requiring oral or IV medications or surgery	1 (0.9%)	3 (2.6%)
Stent obstruction	5 (4.3%)	–
Blur or visual disturbance	4 (3.4%)	8 (6.8%)
Stent malposition	3 (2.6%)	–
Iritis	1 (0.9%)	6 (5.1%)
Conjunctival irritation from hypotensive medication	1 (0.9%)	3 (2.6%)
Disk hemorrhage	1 (0.9%)	3 (2.6%)

Abbreviations: *IOP* intraocular pressure
Data from Craven et al. J Cataract Refract Surg. 2012;38:1339–1345
[a]Corneal edema, anterior chamber cell, corneal abrasion, discomfort, subconjunctival hemorrhage, blurred vision, floaters

Table 3.2 Clinical studies involving single iStent placement in combination with phacoemulsification

Study	Design	n	Follow-up (months)	IOP reduction mmHg (treatment)	IOP reduction mmHg (control)	Medication reduction (treatment)	Medication reduction (control)
Fea [38]	RCT	12	15	3 (17%)	1 (9%)	1.6 (80%)	0.6 (32%)
Samuelson et al. [14]	RCT	111	12	8 (33%)	8 (33%)	1.4 (87%)	1.0 (73%)
Craven et al. [15]	RCT	116	24	8 (33%)	7 (28%)	1.3 (81%)	1.0 (67%)
Spiegel et al. [39]	NRS	48	12	4 (18%)	–	1.2 (75%)	–
Arriola-Villalobos et al. [40]	NRS	19	60	3 (16%)	–	0.5 (36%)	–
Vandewalle et al. [41]	CS	10	12	4 (19%)	–	1.0 (37%)	–
Patel et al. [42]	CS	40	6	4 (21%)	–	1.7 (74%)	–
Neuhann [43]	NRS	62	36	9.2 (36%)	–	1.5 (83%)	–
Ferguson et al. [44]	CS	350	24	3.96 (20.7%)	–	0.58 (49%)	–
Seibold et al. [45]	CS	64	12	1.5 (10.2%)	–	0.4 (22%)	–

Note: The value under medication reduction refers to the decrease in the mean number of hypotensive agents, followed by the mean percent reduction from baseline
Abbreviations: *RCT* randomized clinical trial, *CS* case series, *NRS* non-randomized study, *IOP* intraocular pressure

therapy and may be of benefit in reducing the medication burden [25]. Similarly, the Synergy Trial was a multicenter prospective, post-market, unmasked study conducted in Europe consisting of 99 patients with OAG who underwent implantation of two GTS400 stents as a stand-alone procedure [26]. Patients were on at least two topical ocular hypotensive medications and required additional IOP lowering. Eighty-one percent of subjects achieved IOP $\leq$ 18 mmHg with either a single medication or no medication. Reduction from preoperative medication burden was seen in 86.9% of patients. A summary of completed studies to date is included within Table 3.3.

The iStent *inject* Study Group conducted a large prospective, randomized, single-masked, concurrently controlled, multicenter clinical trial to compare the effect between combined cataract surgery and iStent *inject* implantation with cataract surgery alone [27]. After uncomplicated phacoemulsification, eyes with mild-to-moderate POAG and unmedicated IOP between 21 and 36 mmHg were randomized 3:1 intraoperatively to iStent *inject* implantation (treatment group, $n = 387$) or no stent implantation (control group, $n = 118$). The primary efficacy measure was defined as $\geq$20% reduction in unmedicated diurnal IOP at month 24 and was seen in 75.8% of treatment eyes versus 61.9% of control eyes ($p = 0.005$). The mean reduction in unmedicated diurnal IOP from baselines was greater in treatment eyes than in control eyes (7.0 ± 4.0 mmHg vs. 5.4 ± 3.7 mmHg, $p < 0.001$). Month 24 medication-free diurnal IOP $\leq$ 18 mmHg was achieved by 63.2% of treatment eyes compared with 50.0% of control eyes (difference 13.2%, 95% confidence interval 2.9–23.4). The safety profile of the treatment group was favorable and similar to that in the control group throughout the 2-year follow-up.

At this time, there have been no studies directly comparing the first- and second-generation iStent models. Glaukos has also launched the iStent *inject* W in Europe in 2020, which is a slight modification of the iStent *inject* with a wide flange at its base, allowing for enhanced visualization during implantation. In addition, the wider flange of the iStent *inject* W improves the predictability of the surgery, by minimizing the risk of "over-implanting" the device which results in the inlet being occluded by trabecular tissue.

3.5   Off-Label Use

Currently, the iStent is approved for use in combination with cataract extraction in the United States, but is licensed for standalone use in Europe. As described previously, Bahler et al. found that the implantation of more than one stent into the canal of cultured human anterior segments provided additional pressure lowering to that achieved with a single stent, but to a lesser degree [10]. Several studies and case reports have since been published demonstrating the efficacy of implanting multiple stents [28–32]. Most notably, Katz et al. conducted a prospective, randomized study of one, two, or three trabecular bypass stents in patients with open-angle glaucoma on topical hypotensive medication [33]. Stent placement was performed as a stand-alone procedure in either phakic or pseudophakic eyes. The initial results were

Table 3.3 Summary of additional trabecular micro-bypass clinical studies

Study	Design	Procedure	n	Follow-up (months)	IOP reduction mmHg (treatment)	IOP reduction mmHg (control)	Medication reduction (treatment)	Medication reduction (control)
Multiple stents								
Fernandez-Barrientos et al. [46]	RCT	Phaco + 2 stents	17	12	7 (27%)	4 (16%)	1.1 (100%)	0.5 (42%)
Belovay et al. [21]	NRS	Phaco + 2–3 stents	53	12	4 (20%)	–	2.0 (74%)	–
iStent alone								
Spiegel et al. [47]	CS	1 stent	6	12	5 (25%)	–	19%	–
Buchacra et al. [48]	NRS	1 stent	10	12	7 (27%)	–	1.1 (62%)	–
Ahmed et al. [31]	NRS	2 stents + travoprost	39	18	10 (47%)	–	1.0 (50%)	–
Katz et al. [33]	RCT	1–3 stents	119	18	1: 10.1 (40.4%) 2: 11.4 (45.6%) 3: 12.4 (49.4%)	–	Decrease of mean IOP shown for patients without medication	–
Donnenfeld et al. [49]	NRS	2 stents	76	36	8.9 (36.9%)	–	89.7% not requiring medication	–
iStent inject								
Fea et al. [25]	RCT	2 stents	94	12	8 (38%)	8 (36%)	N/A[a]	N/A[a]
Arriola-Villalobos et al. [50]	CS	Phaco + 1–2 stents	20	12	9 (36%)	–	1.0 (77%)	–
Voskanyan et al. [26]	NRS	2 stents	99	12	10 (40%)	–	71.7% not requiring medication	–
Klamann et al. [28]	CS	2 stents	35	6	POAG: 7.0 (33.0%) PXG: 8.42 (35.5%)	–	POAG: 1.31 (60%) PXG: 1.29 (55%)	–
Arriola-Villalobos et al. [51]	CS	Phaco + 2 stents	20	47 (mean)	9.74 (36.9%)	–	0.55 (42%)	–

Note: The value under medication reduction refers to the decrease in the mean number of hypotensive agents, followed by the mean percent reduction from baseline

Abbreviations: *RCT* randomized clinical trial, *CS* case series, *NRS* non-randomized study, *IOP* intraocular pressure, *phaco* phacoemulsification, *POAG* primary open-angle glaucoma, *PXG* pseudoexfoliative glaucoma

[a]Medical therapy control group

reported in 2015 with a total of 38 subjects receiving 1 stent, 41 subjects with 2 stents, and 40 with 3 stents. They were randomly assigned with a postmedication-washout baseline IOP ranging between 22 and 38. At 18 months, unmedicated mean IOP was 15.9 ± 0.9 with 1 stent, 14.1 ± 1.0 with 2 stents, and 12.2 ± 1.1 with 3 stents. Both the IOP reduction and decrease in medication use were found to be significantly greater with each additional stent. In 2018, the 42-month outcomes were reported [34]. By comparison, month 12 saw IOP reduction $\geq 20\%$ without medication achieved in 89, 90, and 92% or one-, two-, and three-stent eyes, respectively; whereas month 42 showed the same reduction in 61, 91, and 91% of eyes. Based on the data available thus far, the additional reduction in both IOP and topical ocular hypotensive use seen with multiple stent implantation shows promise for iStent use in patients with more advanced disease and further prospective study is warranted. In addition, potential long-term health resource use may be reduced with the improved IOP control achieved with multiple stent placement versus more traditional treatment modalities such as selective laser trabeculoplasty or topical medications [35].

iStent implantation in phakic patients and after previous filtering surgery has also been evaluated [30, 31]. A prospective study by Ahmed et al. involved 39 phakic patients with unmedicated baseline IOP between 22 and 38 mmHg. Patients received two stents placed through a clear corneal incision. The mean unmedicated IOP decreased from 25.3 ± 1.8 mmHg preoperatively to 17.1 ± 2.2 mmHg at 13 months postoperatively [31]. Ferguson et al. inserted a single iStent in a retrospective series of 42 pseudophakic eyes. Medication use was reduced or unchanged in 80% of patients at 1 year, although not of statistical significance. In addition, mean IOP at 2 years was noted to improve from 20.26 ± 6.00 mmHg to 13.62 ± 4.55 ($p < 0.01$) [36].

Angle closure is currently a contraindication for iStent implantation. At present, only one prospective study has evaluated the safety and efficacy of iStent implantation in angle-closure eyes. Hernstadt et al. showed that the mean postoperative IOP decreased from 17.5 ± 3.8 mmHg to 14.8 ± 3.9 mmHg in 37 eyes with angle-closure disease 1 year after combined iStent trabecular micro-bypass device and phacoemulsification ($p < 0.001$). There were no sight-threatening intraoperative or postoperative complications reported, but iStent occlusion with iris occurred in 27% of eyes [37]. However, it was not possible to determine the additional effect of iStent implantation in lowering the IOP compared with phacoemulsification alone. A randomized study comparing phacoemulsification alone with the combined procedure in angle-closure eyes showed that the combined procedure was associated with a higher likelihood of complete success (87.5% [95% CI 58.6-96.7%] vs 43.8% [95% CI 19.8-65.6%]) [52].

A summary of additional trabecular micro-bypass clinical studies to date is demonstrated in Table 3.3 and illustrates the efficacy of iStent alone, multiple stents, as well as the previously discussed iStent *inject*.

3.6   Conclusion

Treating glaucoma patients has traditionally consisted of medications, laser, or filtering surgery. The well-known complications that may accompany trabeculectomy or tube shunt placement have led to the development of new therapeutic approaches including the iStent and iStent *inject* implants. Although the reduction in intraocular pressure seen with these devices is not comparable to filtering surgery, a majority of patients can expect additional improvement versus cataract surgery alone. Another added benefit is seen in the potential reduction of ocular hypotensive medication dependency. As new long-term data become available, indications may expand to certain types of secondary glaucoma, use without concomitant phacoemulsification, and more advanced disease. Among minimally invasive glaucoma surgeries, the iStent currently provides a promising benefit for mild–moderate open-angle glaucoma patients with a favorable safety profile and sparing of conjunctival tissue should more aggressive intervention be necessary in the future.

References

1. Okeke CO, Quigley HA, Jampel HD, et al. Adherence with topical glaucoma medication monitored electronically the Travatan Dosing Aid study. Ophthalmology. 2009;116:191–9.
2. Karmel M. Glaucoma treatment paradigm driven by new interventions. EyeNet Magazine. 2011:41–5.
3. Francis BA, Singh K, Lin SC, et al. Novel glaucoma procedures: a report by the American Academy of Ophthalmology. Ophthalmology. 2011;118:1466–80.
4. Rosenquist R, Epstein D, Melamed S, Johnson M, Grant WM. Outflow resistance of enucleated human eyes at two different perfusion pressures and different extents of trabeculotomy. Curr Eye Res. 1989;8(12):1233–40.
5. Zeimer RC, Gieser DK, Wilensky JT, Noth JM, Mori MM, Odunukwe EE. A practical venomanometer. Measurement of episcleral venous pressure and assessment of the normal range. Arch Ophthalmol. 1983;101(9):1447–9.
6. Toris CB, Yablonski ME, Wang WL, Camras CB. Humor dynamics in the aging human eye. Am J Ophthalmol. 1999;127(4):407–12.
7. Sultan M, Blondeau P. Episcleral venous pressure in younger and older subjects in the sitting and supine positions. J Glaucoma. 2003;12(4):370–3.
8. Selbach JM, Posielek K, Steuhl KP, Kremmer S. Episcleral venous pressure in untreated primary open-angle and normal-tension glaucoma. Ophthalmologica. 2005;219(6):357–61.
9. Zhou J, Smedley GT. A trabecular bypass flow hypothesis. J Glaucoma. 2005;14:74–83.
10. Bahler CK, Smedley GT, Zhou J, Johnson DH. Trabecular bypass stents decrease intraocular pressure in cultured human anterior segments. Am J Ophthalmol. 2004;138:988–94.
11. Bahler CK, Hann CR, Fjield T, Haffner D, Heitzmann H, Fautsch MP. Second-generation trabecular meshwork bypass stent (iStent inject) increases outflow facility in cultured human anterior segments. Am J Ophthalmol. 2012;153:1206–13.
12. Karmel M. Two approaches to MIGS: iStent and trabectome. EyeNet Magazine. 2014:36–41.
13. Zheng CX, Moster MR, Gogte P, Dai Y, Manzi RS, Waisbourd M. Implantation of trabecular micro-bypass stent using a novel "landing strip" technique. Int J Ophthalmol. 2017;10(5):738–41.
14. Samuelson TW, Katz LJ, Wells JM, Duh Y, Giamporcaro JE. Randomized evaluation of the trabecular micro-bypass stent with phacoemulsification in patients with glaucoma and cataract. Ophthalmology. 2011;118:459–67.
15. Craven ER, Katz LJ, Wells JM, Giamporcaro JE. Cataract surgery with trabecular micro-bypass stent implantation in patients with mild-to-moderate open-angle glaucoma and cataract: two-year follow-up. J Cataract Refract Surg. 2012;38:1339–45.

16. Sandhu S, Arora S, Edwards MC. A case of delayed-onset recurrent hyphema after iStent surgery. Can J Ophthalmol. 2016;51:e165–7.
17. Mantravadi AV, Lin C, Kinariwala B, Waisbourd M. Inadvertent implantation of an iStent in the supraciliary space identified by ultrasound biomicroscopy. Can J Ophthalmol. 2016;51:e167–8.
18. Fellman RL, Grover DS. Episcleral venous fluid wave: intraoperative evidence for patency of the conventional outflow system. J Glaucoma. 2014;23(6):347–50.
19. Fellman RL, Feuer MS, Grover DS. Episcleral venous fluid wave correlates with trabectome outcomes. Ophthalmology. 2015;122(12):2385–91.
20. Hann CR, Fautsch MP. Preferential fluid flow in the human trabecular meshwork near collector channels. Invest Ophthalmol Vis Sci. 2009;50(4):1692–7.
21. Belovay GW, Naqi A, Chan BJ, Rateb M, Ahmed IIK. Using multiple trabecular micro-bypass stents in cataract patients to treat open-angle glaucoma. J Cataract Refract Surg. 2012;38:1911–7.
22. Augustinus CJ, Zeyen T. The effect of phacoemulsification and combined phaco/glaucoma procedures on the intraocular pressure in open-angle glaucoma. A review of the literature. Bull Soc Belge Ophtalmol. 2012;320:51–66.
23. Le K, Saheb H. iStent trabecular micro-bypass stent for open-angle glaucoma. Clin Ophthalmol. 2014;8:1937–45.
24. Wellik SR, Dale EA. A review of the iStent trabecular micro-bypass stent: safety and efficacy. Clin Ophthalmol. 2015;9:677–84.
25. Fea AM, Belda JI, Rekas M, et al. Prospective unmasked randomized evaluation of the iStent inject versus two ocular hypotensive agents in patients with primary open-angle glaucoma. Clin Ophthalmol. 2014;8:875–82.
26. Voskanyan L, Garcia-Feijoo J, Belda JI, Fea A, Junemann A, Baudouin C. Prospective, unmasked evaluation of the iStent inject system for open-angle glaucoma: synergy trial. Adv Ther. 2014;31(2):189–201.
27. Samuelson TW, Sarkisian SR Jr, Lubeck D, et al. Prospective, randomized, controlled pivotal trial of iStent inject trabecular micro-bypass in primary open-angle glaucoma and cataract: two-year results. Ophthalmology. 2019;126:811–21.
28. Klamann M, Gonnermann J, Pahlitzsch M, et al. iStent inject in phakic open angle glaucoma. Graefes Arch Clin Exp Ophthalmol. 2015;253(6):941–7.
29. Karmel M. Two approaches to MIGS: iStent and trabectome. EyeNet Magazine. 2014:36–41.
30. Roelofs K, Arora S, Dorey MW. Implantation of 2 trabecular microbypass stents in a patient with primary open-angle glaucoma refractory to previous glaucoma-filtering surgeries. J Cataract Refract Surg. 2014;40:1322–4.
31. Ahmed IIK, Katz LJ, Chang DF, et al. Prospective evaluation of microinvasive glaucoma surgery with trabecular microbypass stents and prostaglandin in open-angle glaucoma. J Cataract Refract Surg. 2014;40:1295–300.
32. Shiba D, Hosoda S, Yaguchi S, Ozeki N, Yuki K, Tsubota K. Safety and efficacy or two trabecular micro-bypass stents as the sole procedure in Japanese patients with medically uncontrolled primary open-angle glaucoma: a pilot case series. J Ophthalmol. 2017;2017:9605461.
33. Katz LJ, Erb C, Carceller GA, Fea AM, Voskanyan L, Wells JM, Giamporcaro JE. Prospective, randomized study of one, two, or three trabecular bypass stents in open-angle glaucoma subjects on topical hypotensive medication. Clin Ophthalmol. 2015;9:2313–20.
34. Katz LJ, Erb C, Carceller GA, Fea AM, Voskanyan L, Giamporcaro JE, Hornbeak DM. Long-term titrated IOP control with one, two, or three trabecular micro-bypass stents in open-angle glaucoma subjects on topical hypotensive medication: 42-month outcomes. Clin Ophthalmol. 2018;12:255–62.
35. Berdahl JP, Khatana AK, Katz LJ, Herndon L, Layton AJ, Yu TM, Bauer MJ, Cantor LB. Cost-comparison of two trabecular micro-bypass stents versus selective laser trabeculoplasty or medications only for intraocular pressure control for patients with open-angle glaucoma. J Med Econ. 2017;20:760–6.

36. Ferguson TJ, Berdahl JP, Schweitzer JA, Sudhagoni R. Evaluation of a trabecular micro-bypass stent in pseudophakic patients with open-angle glaucoma. J Glaucoma. 2016;25(11):896–900.
37. Hernstadt DJ, Cheng J, Htoon HM, et al. Case series of combined iStent implantation and phacoemulsification in eyes with primary angle closure disease: one-year outcomes. Adv Ther. 2019;36:976–86.
38. Fea AM. Phacoemulsification versus phacoemulsification with micro-bypass stent implantation in primary open-angle glaucoma: randomized double-masked clinical trial. J Cataract Refract Surg. 2010;36(3):407–12.
39. Spiegel D, Wetzel W, Neuhann T, et al. Coexistent primary open-angle glaucoma and cataract: interim analysis of a trabecular micro-bypass stent and concurrent cataract surgery. Eur J Ophthalmol. 2009;19(3):393–9.
40. Arriola-Villalobos P, Martínez-de-la-Casa JM, Díaz-Valle D, Fernández-Pérez C, García-Sánchez J, García-Feijoó J. Combined iStent trabecular micro-bypass stent implantation and phacoemulsification for coexistent open-angle glaucoma and cataract: a long-term study. Br J Ophthalmol. 2012;96(5):645–9.
41. Vandewalle E, Zeyen T, Stalmans I. The iStent trabecular micro-bypass stent: a case series. Bull Soc Belge Ophtalmol. 2009;311:23–9.
42. Patel I, de Klerk TA, Au L. Manchester iStent study: early results from a prospective UK case series. Clin Exp Ophthalmol. 2013;41(7):648–52.
43. Neuhann TH. Trabecular micro-bypass stent implantation during small-incision cataract surgery for open-angle glaucoma or ocular hypertension: long-term results. J Cataract Refract Surg. 2015;41(12):2664–71.
44. Ferguson TJ, Berdahl JP, Schweitzer JA, Sudhagoni R. Clinical evaluation of a trabecular microbypass stent with phacoemulsification in patients with open-angle glaucoma and cataract. Clin Ophthalmol. 2016;10:1767–73.
45. Seibold LK, Garnett KM, Kennedy JB, et al. Outcomes after combined phacoemulsification and trabecular microbypass stent implantation in controlled open-angle glaucoma. J Cataract Refract Surg. 2016;42(9):1332–8.
46. Fernandez-Barrientos Y, Garcia-Feijoo J, Martinez-de-la-Casa JM, Pablo LE, Fernandez-Perez C, Garcia SJ. Fluorophotometric study of the effect of the glaukos trabecular microbypass stent on aqueous humor dynamics. Invest Ophthalmol Vis Sci. 2010;51(7):3327–32.
47. Spiegel D, Wetzel W, Haffner DS, Hill RA. Initial clinical experience with the trabecular micro-bypass stent in patients with glaucoma. Adv Ther. 2007;24(1):161–70.
48. Buchacra O, Duch S, Milla E, Stirbu O. One-year analysis of the iStent trabecular microbypass in secondary glaucoma. Clin Ophthalmol. 2011;5:321–6.
49. Donnenfeld ED, Solomon KD, Voskanyan L, et al. A prospective 3-year follow-up trial of implantation of two trabecular microbypass in open-angle glaucoma. Clin Ophthalmol. 2015;9:2057–65.
50. Arriola-Villalobos P, Martinez-de-la-Casa JM, Diaz-Valle D, et al. Mid-term evaluation of the new Glaukos iStent with phacoemulsification in coexistent open-angle glaucoma or ocular hypertension and cataract. Br J Ophthalmol. 2013;97(10):1250–5.
51. Arriola-Villalobos P, Martinez-de-la-Casa JM, Diaz-Valle D, et al. Glaukos iStent inject trabecular micro-bypass implantation associated with cataract surgery in patients with coexisting cataract and open-angle glaucoma or ocular hypertension: a long-term study. J Ophthalmol. 2016;2016:1–7.
52. Chen DZ, Sng CCA, Sangtam T, et al. Phacoemulsification vs phacoemulsification with micro-bypass stent implantation in primary angle closure and primary angle closure glaucoma: A randomized single-masked clinical study. Clin Exp Ophthalmol. 2020;48(4):450–61.

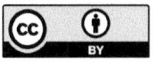

Ab-Interno Trabeculotomy

4

Richard L. Rabin, Jaehong Han, and Douglas J. Rhee

4.1   Introduction

Multiple experimental and morphological studies of primate and human eyes have demonstrated that the anatomical location of the greatest resistance to aqueous outflow is at the juxtacanalicular trabecular meshwork [1, 2]. To overcome this resistance, goniotomy was first introduced in 1936 as the first surgical procedure directed at the trabecular meshwork, with significant success in infants and young children with congenital glaucoma, but relatively poor outcomes in adults [3]. Opening Schlemm's canal to direct aqueous outflow can be accomplished in adults from either an *ab-externo* or an *ab-interno* approach. In 1989, Rosenquist et al. studied the aqueous outflow resistance of enucleated human eyes and showed that complete (12 clock hours) internal trabeculotomy reduced 71% of the aqueous outflow resistance in eyes with 25 mmHg intraocular pressure. They also reported that with just one clock hour of trabeculotomy, 41% of the total effect was obtained [4].

Trabectome (NeoMedix Corporation, San Juan Capistrano, CA, USA) received approval by the US Food and Drug Administration in April 2004. The first published trial of US patients was in January 2006 for the surgical treatment of open-angle glaucoma. The Trabectome removes a segment of the trabecular meshwork and the inner wall of the Schlemm's canal using an *ab-interno* approach, enhancing aqueous outflow via increased access to the Schlemm's canal and the collector channels (Fig. 4.1).

R. L. Rabin · J. Han · D. J. Rhee (✉)
Department of Ophthalmology and Visual Sciences, University Hospitals, Cleveland Medical Center, Cleveland, OH, USA

Case Western Reserve University School of Medicine, Cleveland, OH, USA
e-mail: Douglas.Rhee@uhhospitals.org

C. C. A. Sng, K. Barton (eds.), *Minimally Invasive Glaucoma Surgery*,
https://doi.org/10.1007/978-981-15-5632-6_4

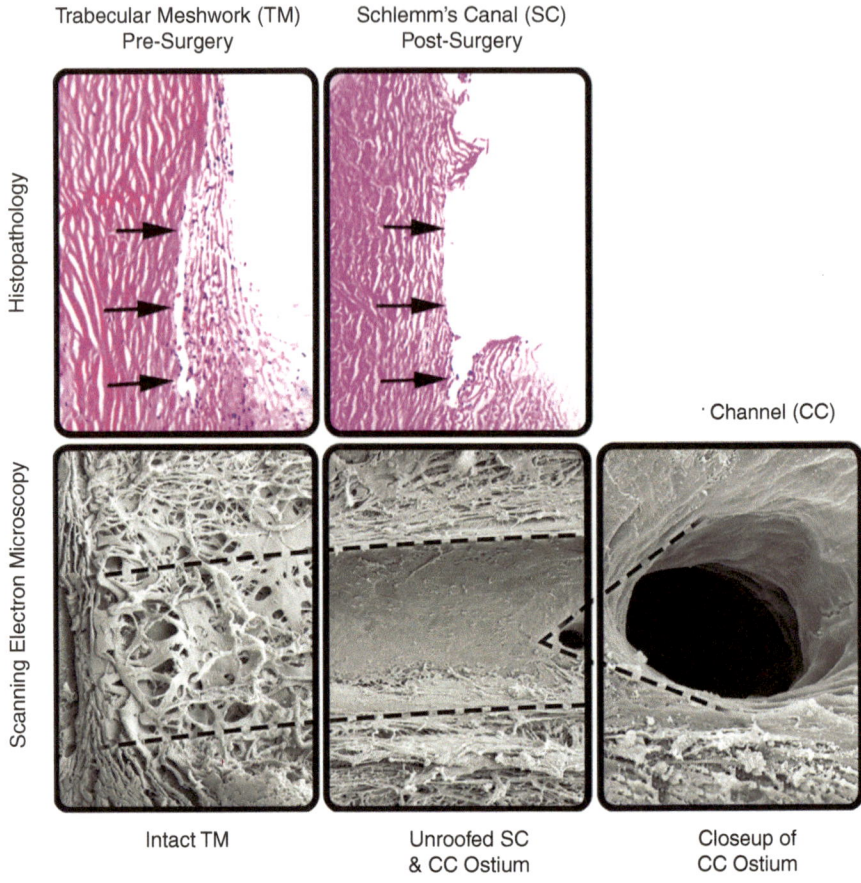

Fig. 4.1 Upper panels: Histopathology images of the trabecular meshwork and Schlemm's canal before and after Trabectome procedure. Lower panels: Electron microscopy images of the anterior chamber angle structures before and after Trabectome procedure. (Copyright NeoMedix Corporation, San Juan Capistrano, CA, USA; reproduced with permission)

4.2   Trabectome Device

The Trabectome device consists of a single-use, disposable handpiece that combines electrocautery, irrigation, and aspiration. The handpiece is connected to a generator with a frequency of 550 kHz that allows adjustments in 0.1 W increments and is controlled via a three-stage foot pedal that initiates irrigation, aspiration, and electrocautery in sequence (Figs. 4.2 and 4.3). Irrigation and aspiration permit removal of debris and regulation of temperature. The tip of the Trabectome is angled at 90° to create a protective triangular-shaped footplate for easier insertion into Schlemm's canal. The footplate is coated permitting smoother movement within the canal and protecting the outer wall of Schlemm's canal from the thermal energy.

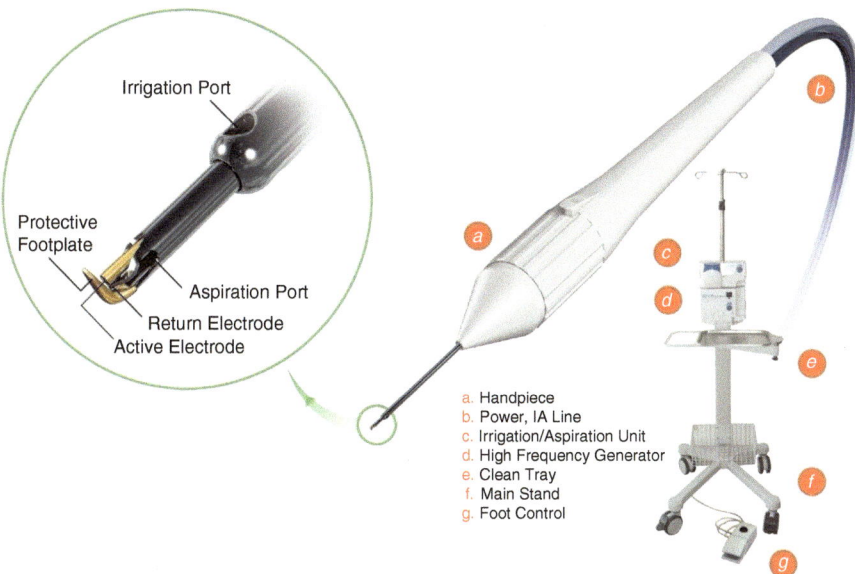

Fig. 4.2 Trabectome console and foot pedal. (Copyright NeoMedix Corporation, San Juan Capistrano, CA, USA; reproduced with permission)

The electrode tip of the Trabectome creates plasma that ablates the trabecular meshwork, thereby creating a less traumatic procedure [5]. Continuous infusion minimizes thermal injury to surrounding structures and aspiration removes tissue debris to allow for more consistent action of the electrode. In studies by Minckler and Francis [6, 7], Trabectome-treated specimens showed less damage to surrounding structures compared to eyes treated by goniotomy blade (Fig. 4.1).

4.3 Trabectome Procedure

Some surgeons pretreat patients with topical apraclonidine 0.5% or brimonidine 0.1% to reduce intraoperative reflux bleeding. Bleeding can also be reduced by adequate pressurization of the anterior chamber at the conclusion of the procedure. The patient's head is tilted 30–45° away from the surgeon and the operating microscope is tilted 30–45° toward the surgeon to create a near 90° viewing angle to the viewing axis of the eye (Fig. 4.3b, c).

When performing both Trabectome and phacoemulsification (phaco-Trabectome), we prefer to perform the Trabectome portion first to optimize corneal clarity. A 1.8 mm, two-step clear corneal incision is created using a keratome blade. The inner third of the incision can be flared to improve mobility of the handpiece and visualization of the surgery by eliminating corneal striae from torquing of the wound. The Trabectome irrigation is activated by depressing the black colored

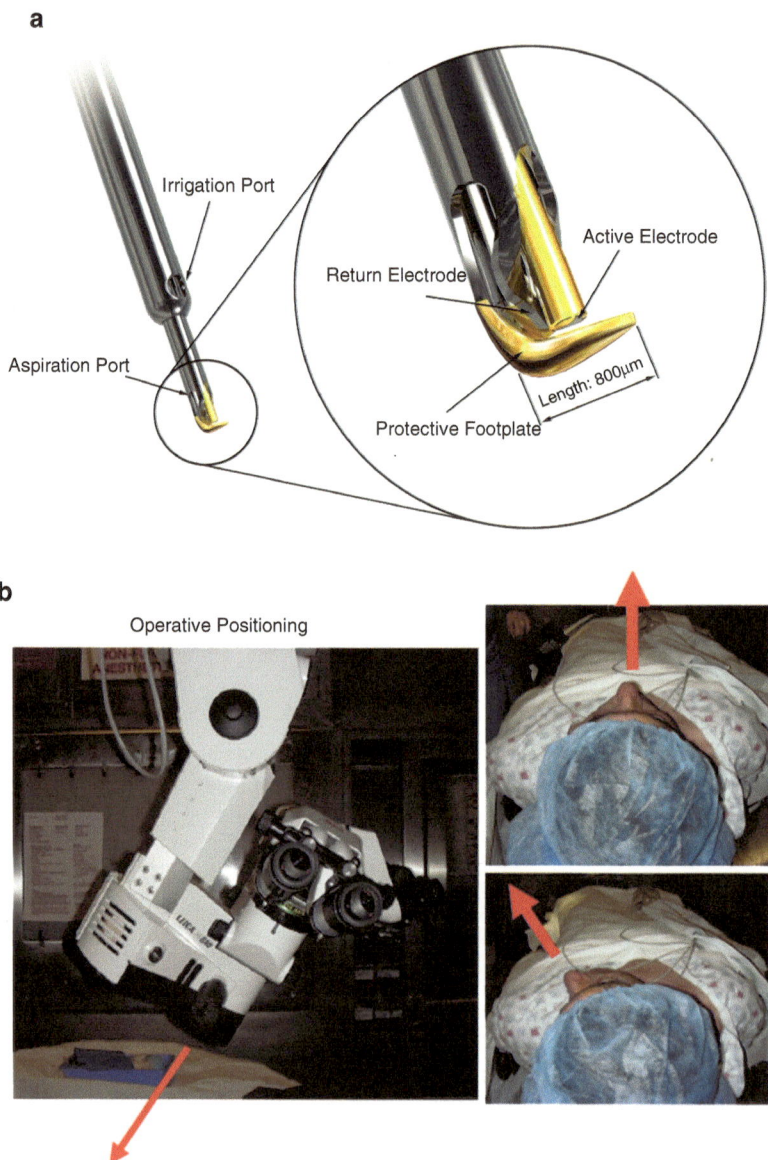

Fig. 4.3 (**a**) Trabectome handpiece distal end: Electrode, aspiration port, and irrigation port are visible. Footplate dimensions: heel to tip, 800 µm; footplate maximum width, 230 µm; footplate maximum thickness, 110 µm. Gap between electrocautery pole and footplate: 150 µm. (Copyright NeoMedix Corporation, San Juan Capistrano, CA, USA; reproduced with permission) (**b**) Microscope and head positioning: Operating room microscope is tilted between 35 and 45° (left panel) while the patient's head is similarly turned 35–45° away from the surgeon. In this example, the patient's position is shown in the typical faceup position for cataract surgery (right upper panel) and appropriate positioning for the right eye for the Trabectome procedure (right lower panel). (**c**) Intraoperative positioning of the operating room microscope and patient's head as shown in **b**. (**d**) Schematic of the centripetal and lateral vectors of motion of the probe while in Schlemm's canal in order to accommodate the circular shape of the canal

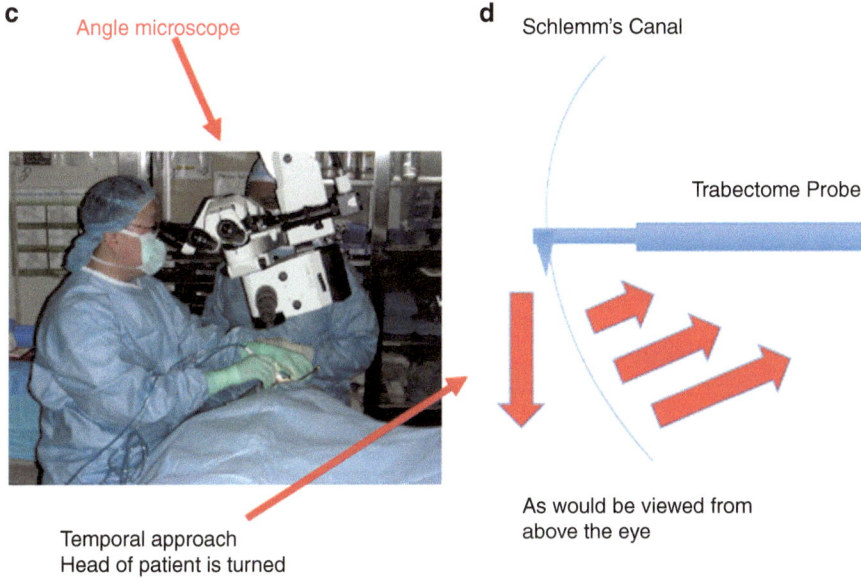

Fig. 4.3 (continued)

button on the foot pedal and the probe is inserted into the anterior chamber under direct visualization. Cohesive viscoelastic (Healon) may be used to deepen the nasal anterior chamber angle and as a coupling agent for the gonioscopy lens. The active irrigation of the Trabectome system helps to keep the anterior chamber formed during the procedure and is designed to reduce the need for viscoelastic in the anterior chamber.

After the probe's irrigation port enters the anterior chamber, the direct view surgical gonioscopy lens, e.g., Swan Jacob gonioprism, is applied on the cornea to view the nasal angle. After the trabecular meshwork is identified, the probe is inserted into Schlemm's canal and the foot pedal is depressed fully to activate aspiration and electrocautery. The foot pedal has three positions—"off" in which neither aspiration nor electrocautery is active, "first position" in which aspiration is active, but not electrocautery, and "second position" in which both aspiration and electrocautery are activated. Torquing of the eye and failure to advance the tip with gentle pressure may indicate that the tip is lodged in the back wall of the Schlemm's canal. This can be corrected by backing the probe up toward the area of previously treated tissue and trying again. During the procedure, it is crucial to eliminate any outward push on Schlemm's canal as this can damage the wall of Schlemm's canal and the collector channel system. It is therefore important to apply a slight inward pull (i.e., toward the pupil) during ablation to offset any tendency to push or rub against the wall of Schlemm's canal (Fig. 4.3d).

After successfully completing one direction of treatment, the Trabectome probe can be rotated 180° and advanced in the opposite direction. Following a successful

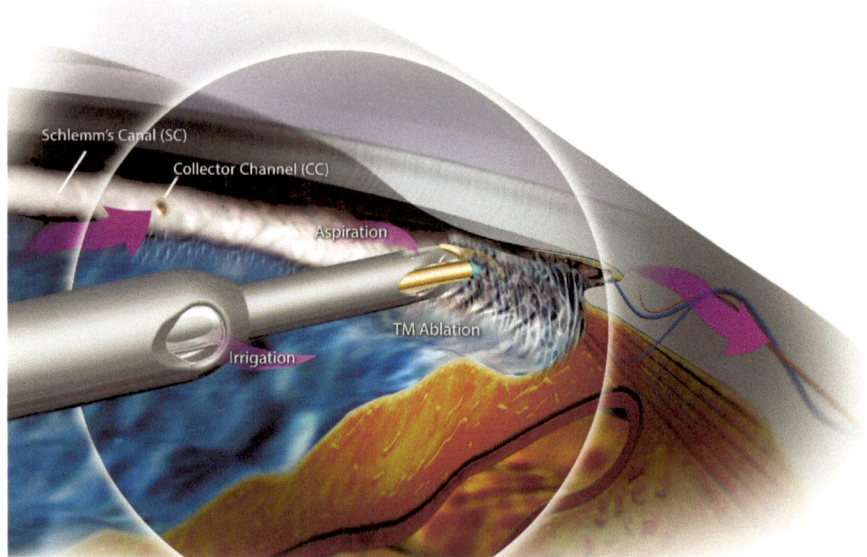

Fig. 4.4 Ablation of trabecular meshwork using the Trabectome probe. (Copyright NeoMedix Corporation, San Juan Capistrano, CA, USA; reproduced with permission)

procedure, the outer wall of Schlemm's canal will appear opalescent (Fig. 4.4). After the treatment, the probe is retracted so that the irrigation port is just inside the wound. The gonioscopy lens is then removed and the probe is removed from the eye under direct visualization. The microscope and patient's head can then be repositioned if cataract surgery is to be performed. A properly constructed wound should seal with stromal hydration.

Most surgeons experienced in Trabectome procedures report treating 60–120° of angle. The length of the ablation arc has not been found to be significantly correlated with the subsequent intraocular pressure (IOP) decrease [8]. Up to 800 mW of electrocautery power can be used. Coagulation necrosis can result if the energy used exceeds 1000 mW, which manifests as darkening along the edge of the ablated tissue.

To reduce intraocular bleeding, air–bubble tamponade in the anterior chamber can be considered or the eye can be pressurized to 20–25 mmHg, provided optic nerve/visual field damage is not advanced and other risk factors for complications associated with transiently elevated IOP are absent, e.g., post-cataract surgery anterior ischaemic optic neuropathy or retinal vascular occlusion following previous eye surgery. Postoperative care generally includes the use of topical antibiotic and steroid eye drops, with a tapering regimen according to the surgeon's preference. In general, we recommend a rapid taper of corticosteroids. Some surgeons advocate prescribing pilocarpine 1–2% postoperatively to prevent the formation of peripheral anterior synechiae.

4.4   Surgical Planning

In patients with mild cataract and glaucoma, many options exist—phacoemulsification alone, minimally invasive glaucoma surgery (MIGS) alone, combined cataract surgery and MIGS, conventional glaucoma surgery, i.e., trabeculectomy and tube shunt implants. The surgery can be either a single operation with multiple procedures performed at the same sitting or staged cataract and glaucoma surgery. Phacoemulsification alone reduces IOP, with the extent of IOP reduction varying between different studies, but is approximately 4 mmHg (16.5%) based on the Ocular Hypertension Treatment Study [9]. This IOP-lowering effect is directly proportional to the IOP prior to surgery. If the patient has a component of angle closure, then cataract removal may be indicated even with 20/20 acuity.

4.4.1   Target IOP

In patients requiring a target IOP below 12 mmHg, Trabectome is not ideal. Devices that are designed to remove or bypass the trabecular meshwork by shunting fluid to Schlemm's canal theoretically cannot achieve IOP below the episcleral venous pressure, 8–10 mmHg [10]. In patients requiring an IOP of 12 mmHg or less, the procedures that may have a higher chance of success create a communication between the anterior chamber and subconjunctival space, e.g., subconjunctival MIGS devices or conventional glaucoma surgery (trabeculectomy, tube shunt device [e.g., Baerveldt or Ahmed glaucoma implant]).

In patients with a target IOP of approximately 15–17 mmHg, Trabectome surgery could be considered. Numerous studies have shown IOP decreases to the 15–17 mmHg range with both phaco-Trabectome and with Trabectome-alone [11–14]. Mizoguchi et al. reported that the Trabectome failure rate was higher in the eyes with a preoperative IOP <18 mmHg and lower in those with a preoperative IOP of 18–22 mmHg [15]. Successful outcomes have been reported in studies with higher baseline IOP as well, such as 37.6 ± 6.6 mmHg in a study by Akil et al. [16] and 31.6 ± 9.9 mmHg by Shoji et al. [17]. These studies suggest that the higher the baseline IOP, the greater the percentage reduction in IOP.

4.4.2   Trabectome Can Be Performed in Patients with Narrow Angles

Trabectome has traditionally been reserved for patients with open angles (at least Shaffer grade 3) because it was thought that the failure rate would increase in patients with narrower angles and that the procedure would be difficult to perform safely. In Trabectome-alone cases and phaco-Trabectome combined cases, Bussel et al. found no significant difference in IOP reduction between eyes with Shaffer grade 3 or greater versus those with grade 2 or less. This would allow many patients who were previously not deemed to be MIGS candidates to be able to benefit from Trabectome [18].

In Chinese patients, Lee et al. reported that despite seeing an open-angle configuration on gonioscopy, the small dimensions of the anterior segment make it difficult to maneuver the Trabectome handpiece in the eye without damaging ocular structures such as the iris. Therefore, they only performed Trabectome surgery on pseudophakic Chinese eyes. Even in pseudophakic Chinese eyes, the view of the treated area of Schlemm's canal was obscured by normal iris (not peripheral anterior synechiae) in some eyes by 1 month after Trabectome surgery, as a consequence of the small anterior segment dimensions. However, this was not correlated with an IOP increase. [19].

4.4.3   Contraindications

Contraindications to trabectome surgery include neovascularization of the anterior chamber angle, glaucoma secondary to elevated episcleral venous pressure, chronic angle closure, and active uveitis [20]. Poor visualization of the trabecular meshwork or a very narrow anterior chamber angle increases the risk of damage to surrounding ocular structures.

4.5   Results of Trabectome

4.5.1   Quality of Evidence

While Trabectome surgery is widely performed, it is important to note the paucity of high-quality evidence. In 2016, Hu et al. conducted a Cochrane review of all published Trabectome studies. They included only randomized controlled trials resulting in the exclusion of all 113 published reports on Trabectome. A single randomized controlled trial was underway, NCT00901108, but has since been terminated [21]. The current compendium of Trabectome literature suffers from a lack of prospective, randomized, controlled studies. Other issues include industry-sponsored studies with poor clinical trial procedures, e.g., enrollment, data collection and methods of patient selection. Variations in surgical techniques are likely to confound the surgical outcomes as each surgeon will ablate a different length of trabecular meshwork.

4.5.2   Clinical Efficacy

4.5.2.1 Trabectome-Alone
In 2005, the first clinical study by Minckler et al. reported results of Trabectome-alone in 15 patients with primary and secondary open-angle glaucoma, who were recruited from a clinical practice in Tijuana, Mexico. At 1 year, the IOP decreased from 22.6 ± 4.7 mmHg to 16.3 ± 2.0 mmHg, with a reduction in the mean number of medications from 1.2 to 0.1 [22].

Table 4.1 Commonly used Success and Failure criteria

Success criterion: postoperative IOP <21 mmHg and reduction of IOP ≥20% from baseline. Failure was determined if these criteria were not met on two consecutive visits after postoperative month 3
Failure: success criterion not met and/or need for additional glaucoma surgery

The largest data set comes from the global Trabectome study database sponsored by the device manufacturer, NeoMedix, which analyzes the first 20 cases of any Trabectome surgeon who voluntarily sends in de-identified clinical data as post-market surveillance. This database is stored by the company, and the most recent update was published in 2014, which included 5435 cases of Trabectome-alone and phaco-Trabectome procedures, with up to 90 months of follow-up. On average, the IOP was reduced from 23.0 ± 7.9 mmHg to 16.5 ± 3.8 mmHg (29% reduction) and the number of glaucoma medications was reduced from 2.6 ± 1.3 to 1.6 ± 1.3 (38%) [23]. However, a large number of patients were lost to follow-up with incomplete data from the first postoperative day, hence limiting the generalizability of these results.

In 2008, Minckler et al. published a follow-up study to update their results [13]. They adapted the success criteria from the Tube versus Trabeculectomy Study to evaluate Trabectome surgery (Table 4.1). This criteria has been adopted by most subsequent Trabectome studies. Although Minckler et al. noted the success rate of Trabectome after 12 months to be 50%, the 1-year success rates have varied significantly in different studies, ranging from 36% [24] to 94% [25]. The study which reported a 1-year success rate of 36% found that this decreased to 22.4% by 2 years [24]. In many of the aforementioned studies, the high dropout rates are likely to introduce selection bias, limiting the generalizability of the study results.

These studies use Kaplan-Meier survival plots to display the success rate over time. The significance of the plots is difficult to interpret because most of the Kaplan-Meier survival plots only show the success rate, but do not indicate the number of patients at each follow-up visit [23]. Inter-study results may vary as a consequence of different study designs, surgical technique, population differences between study groups, or different patient evaluation protocols (e.g., masked vs. unmasked IOP readings) [6–8, 11, 15–17, 22–24, 26].

4.5.2.2 Trabectome-Alone Versus Trabeculectomy with Mitomycin C

In a retrospective cohort study, Jea et al. compared Trabectome to trabeculectomy with mitomycin C. This cohort study had a very low rate of participant dropout. After 24 months, IOP decreased from 28.1 ± 8.6 mmHg to 15.9 ± 4.5 mmHg in the Trabectome group versus 26.3 ± 10.9 mmHg to 10.2 ± 4.1 mmHg in the trabeculectomy group; 43.5% of Trabectome eyes and 10.8% of trabeculectomy eyes required subsequent glaucoma surgery. Two-year success rates were 22.4% and 76.1% in the Trabectome and trabeculectomy groups respectively, demonstrating a lower success rate of Trabectome compared to trabeculectomy. Younger age and lower preoperative IOP were risk factors for Trabectome failure [24]. The results were later corroborated by Sit et al. [27].

4.5.2.3 Phaco-Trabectome Versus Trabectome-Alone

Neiweem et al. published an algorithm to calculate anticipated IOP after Trabectome. They found that phacoemulsification plays a minimal role in IOP reduction when performed with Trabectome surgery. They calculated that adding phacoemulsification to Trabectome surgery lowers final IOP by only 0.73 ± 0.32 mmHg [28]. Similarly, studies have shown that there is no significant difference in the mean postoperative IOP and the mean number of hypotensive medications for phaco-Trabectome compared with Trabectome-alone [23, 25]. However, these findings are contradictory to the results of randomized control trials comparing cataract surgery alone to cataract surgery combined with other MIGS procedures, including iStent, CyPass, and Hydrus implantation.

Other studies have reported that the success rate of phaco-Trabectome is higher than that of Trabectome-alone. In a meta-analysis by Kapowitz et al., the mean 1-year success rate of Trabectome-alone was $61 \pm 17\%$ ($n = 5$ studies) and that of phaco-Trabectome was $85 \pm 17\%$ ($n = 6$ studies) [29].

4.5.3   Phaco-Trabectome Versus Phaco-iStent

Three nonrandomized retrospective studies have compared phaco-Trabectome to phacoemulsification with two iStents [12–14]. In all three studies, there were no statistical differences between the postoperative IOP and the number of medications between the two groups. Lavia et al. came to the same conclusion in a meta-analysis [30].

4.5.4   Preoperative Glaucoma Severity on Surgical Outcome

It is thought that MIGS is most effective for mild-to-moderate glaucoma. Roy et al. looked at the 1-year postoperative outcomes of 498 patients undergoing phaco-Trabectome, and stratified results based on a pre-operative glaucoma severity index which incorporated pre-operative IOP, the number of hypotensive medications and visual field status. Severity was designated on a scale of 1 through 4 with a higher number indicating more severe disease. Success rates after 1 year were noted to be 98, 93, 96, and 88% in groups 1 to 4 respectively, with a 1.69 ± 0.2 mmHg larger IOP reduction with each increase in group number. This study suggests that phaco-Trabectome surgery can be successful for severe glaucoma in carefully selected patients [31], though the efficacy of conventional glaucoma surgery (trabeculectomy and tube shunt implants) is certainly much more established in such patients.

4.5.5   Other Potential Factors Affecting Efficacy

4.5.5.1 Does Prior Ineffective Selective Laser Trabeculoplasty (SLT) Alter Trabectome Outcomes?

Vold et al. retrospectively compared the impact of Trabectome surgery on patients with and without prior SLT treatment [32]. No significant difference in IOP was found between the two groups. At 1 year, patients without prior SLT treatment

($n = 177$) had mean IOP of 16.5 ± 4.0 mmHg, while those with prior SLT treatment ($n = 58$) had mean IOP of 15.7 ± 3.0 mmHg.

Klamann et al. retrospectively compared the 6-month outcomes of eyes which underwent combined phaco-Trabectome 3 months after 360° SLT, compared with eyes which did not undergo prior SLT. In eyes with POAG, there was no significant difference in IOP between the two groups at 6 months. In eyes with pigment dispersion and pseudoexfoliation, those that underwent prior SLT had a greater IOP reduction compared with those without previous SLT, though this difference was significant only at the 6-month time point and the number of hypotensive medications was similar between the two groups. In view of the small sample size, the lack of masking and a significant difference between the two groups being detectable only at a single time point, these results must be verified in a larger study before extrapolation to clinical practice [33].

4.5.5.2 Trabectome for Patients with Secondary Open-Angle Glaucoma

Pseudoexfoliation glaucoma, pigmentary glaucoma, and steroid-induced glaucoma have responded well to Trabectome surgery [26, 33–35]. Pahlitzsch et al. compared Trabectome-alone in POAG versus pseudoexfoliation glaucoma patients. They showed an IOP reduction from 19.10 ± 4.11 mmHg to 14.27 ± 2.93 mmHg and glaucoma medication reduction from 2.40 ± 0.92 to 1.77 ± 1.00 in the POAG group after 36 months. The pseudoexfoliation group had an IOP decrease from 22.49 ± 9.40 mmHg to 14.57 ± 5.05 mmHg and glaucoma medication reduction from 2.31 ± 1.02 to 1.75 ± 0.91 after 36 months [26]. Steroid-induced glaucoma has also responded well to Trabectome surgery [34, 35]. Dang et al. showed that the success rates were 86% and 85% respectively for steroid-induced glaucoma and POAG at 1-year follow-up [34]. Trabectome surgery has been shown to be effective in uveitic glaucoma as well [36].

Some studies suggest that Trabectome surgery may be more successful in secondary open-angle glaucoma (SOAG) compared to POAG. In a Japanese study by Shoji et al., the success rate at 12 months for POAG patients ($n = 80$) and SOAG patients ($n = 46$) were $53.9 \pm 7.5\%$ and $77.2 \pm 5.4\%$, respectively [17]. In the SOAG group, 11 patients had steroid-induced glaucoma, 22 patients had pseudoexfoliation glaucoma, and 13 patients had uveitic glaucoma. In a study by Ting et al., success rates at 12 months for POAG and pseudoexfoliation glaucoma patients were 62.9 and 79.1% respectively ($P = 0.004$) [37]. Akil et al. found that Trabectome-alone success rates after 12 months were 86 and 92% for POAG and pigmentary glaucoma patients, respectively [16].

It is believed that Trabectome works well for secondary open-angle glaucoma, in particular pseudoexfoliation glaucoma and pigmentary glaucoma, because the site of greatest aqueous outflow resistance is at the trabecular meshwork (due to occlusion by pseudoexfoliative material or pigment), hence these eyes should respond well to trabecular meshwork removal.

4.5.5.3 Trabectome Can Be Performed in Patients with Previous Failed Trabeculectomy

It was previously believed that following conventional glaucoma surgery, aqueous flow through the trabecular outflow pathway decreased significantly. Bussel et al. showed that Trabectome surgery can be beneficial with or without phacoemulsification in eyes with failed trabeculectomy [38]. At 1 year postoperatively, the mean IOP of the Trabectome-only group decreased by 28% from a baseline of 23.7 mmHg while that of the phaco-Trabectome group decreased by 19% from a baseline of 20 mmHg. The mean number of hypotensive medications decreased from 2.8 to 2.0 in the Trabectome-only group and from 2.5 to 1.6 in the phaco-Trabectome group.

4.5.5.4 Intraoperative Prognosticator for Postoperative Outcome

Fellman et al. suggested that a prominent post-Trabectome episcleral venous fluid wave may be a reliable biomarker for successful Trabectome surgery [39]. Immediately after the Trabectome procedure, the extent of episcleral venous blanching adjacent to the Trabectome site was noted in response to increased IOP, achieved by adjusting the irrigation level within the anterior chamber. Preoperatively, patients had mean IOP of 19.3 ± 5.1 mmHg on 2.7 ± 0.9 medications. Patients with a prominent fluid wave had a post-Trabectome mean IOP of 13.3 ± 2.7 mmHg on 1.4 ± 1.2 medications while patients with a poor fluid wave had a post-Trabectome mean IOP of 18.4 ± 3.1 mmHg on 2.9 ± 0.9 medications at 12 months follow-up. However, the study did not report the preoperative IOP and number of medications separately for the two cohorts, hence it was possible that the difference in postoperative outcomes between the groups might be partly attributable to preoperative differences. A reliable method of assessing the preoperative episcleral venous flow has not been established and the magnitude of increase in episcleral venous flow secondary to Trabectome surgery is unclear. Furthermore, the value of this sign for preoperative prognostication is limited as it can only be observed after the procedure has been performed.

4.6 Complications of Trabectome

In 2008, Minckler et al. reported the rate of complications associated with Trabectome surgery from a review of 1127 patients [40]. In this study, 17 patients (1.5%) had hypotony (IOP < 5 mmHg) at day 1, 65 patients (5.8%) had an IOP spike (IOP >10 mmHh above baseline), 874 patients (77.6%) had intraoperative blood reflux, and one patient had aqueous misdirection (0.09%). Infection, wound leak, bleb formation, choroidal effusion, choroidal hemorrhage, or visual acuity decrease of more than two lines did not occur in any of the patients [40] (Table 4.2).

In the study by Francis et al. which included 304 eyes that underwent phaco-Trabectome, an IOP spike of 10 mmHg or greater occurred in 26 eyes (8.6%) at day 1 and in 6 eyes (2.0%) at week 1 after the surgery. Francis et al. also noted minor iris injury from the Trabectome tip in four cases (1.3%) [42].

Mizoguchi et al. reported that the complications after Trabectome surgery included microhyphema (76.8%), hyphema (23.2%), IOP spike >10 mmHg (4.9%), decrease in VA greater than two lines (1.2%), and cataract progression (1.2%) [15].

Table 4.2 Complications of Trabectome surgery	Intraoperative blood reflux (78% of 1127 cases) [40]; 92% of 557 [41]
	Postoperative hyphema (23.2% of 82 cases) [15]
	Peripheral anterior synechiae (14.0% of 101 cases) [6]
	Transient IOP spike (5.8% of 1127 cases) [40]
	IOP at 1 week >10 mmHg higher than preop (2.0% of 304 cases) [42]
	Hypotony (1.5% of 1127 cases) [40]
	Cyclodialysis cleft, low incidence rate [43, 44]
	Iris injury (1.3% of 304 cases) [42]
	Cataract progression (1.2% of 82 cases) [15]

Serious complications are rare after Trabectome surgery, with the incidence similar to that associated with cataract surgery [29]. Maeda et al. showed that there was no statistically significant difference in corneal endothelial cell count before and after Trabectome surgery [45].

The most common reasons for surgical failure are incomplete or improper removal of the trabecular meshwork, ablation of the wrong site hence damaging the ciliary body, and damage to Schlemm's canal or surrounding tissue which results in scarring. While blood reflux from the collector channels is common, surgical intervention for hyphema is rare [46]. Peripheral anterior synechiae have been observed in nearly a quarter of patients in some studies [6].

Berk et al. documented the first case of cyclodialysis cleft secondary to a complicated Trabectome procedure which resulted in hypotony requiring direct suture cyclopexy [43]. While there have been a few reports on cyclodialysis cleft formation after Trabectome surgery, it may be an underreported complication. A cyclodialysis cleft may be difficult to identify in the clinic postoperatively, as the associated hypotony may narrow the anterior chamber angle and hinder visualization of the ciliary body band. Ultrasound biomicroscopy may be helpful in identifying cyclodialysis clefts postoperatively [44]. The cleft is most easily visualized immediately after creation when the eye is still pressurized from the Trabectome infusion.

One should suspect a cleft intraoperatively when there is excessive bleeding or when the postoperative IOP reduction is more than expected. Closure of the cleft typically results in a transient IOP spike which usually lasts about 4–5 days.

4.7   After Trabectome Has Failed

4.7.1   Does Trabectome Surgery Impact Future Glaucoma Surgery Outcomes?

Trabectome surgery spares the conjunctiva and Jea et al. showed that failed Trabectome surgery did not impact the success of subsequent trabeculectomy [47]. However, after failed Trabectome surgery, subsequent SLT has limited benefit [48].

4.7.2 Gonioscopy-Assisted Transluminal Trabeculotomy (GATT) Procedure as a Potential Treatment Option After Failed Trabectome Surgery

GATT is adapted from *ab-externo* trabeculotomy to create a safer and easier approach to access Schlemm's canal. A microcatheter is fed into Schlemm's canal more than 360° using an *ab-interno* approach through a trabecular incision. GATT has been shown to be effective at decreasing medication reliance and improving IOP in both primary and secondary glaucoma [49, 50]. Hyphema is the most frequent complication and is present in 34% of eyes 1 week after the surgery.

In patients who initially responded to Trabectome surgery but subsequently developed elevated IOP again, GATT may be beneficial as it allows aqueous to access a larger segment of Schlemm's canal than Trabectome surgery. The GATT fiber optic probe may be inserted into the Schlemm's canal through the previous Trabectome trabecular incision.

4.8 Conclusion

Trabectome surgery bypasses the trabecular meshwork and allows aqueous to flow directly from the anterior chamber to the Schlemm's canal. This is a bleb-less procedure which spares the conjunctiva. Multiple studies have shown that Trabectome surgery results in a reduction in IOP and the number of ocular hypotensive agents, though the efficacy is significantly less than conventional glaucoma surgery. Trabectome surgery has a favorable safety profile compared with conventional filtration surgery, with the most common complication being intraoperative and postoperative bleeding. Disadvantages of Trabectome surgery include the modest efficacy, which is limited by episcleral venous pressure, and the difficulty in targeting treatment to the segment of Schlemm's canal with the highest concentration of functional collector channels. Additional research is required to understand how the efficacy of Trabectome surgery can be maximized.

References

1. Brubaker RF. Targeting outflow facility in glaucoma management. Surv Ophthalmol. 2003;48(Suppl 1):S17–20.
2. Lutjen-Drecoll E. Functional morphology of the trabecular meshwork in primate eyes. Prog Retin Eye Res. 1999;18(1):91–119.
3. Chihara E, Nishida A, Kodo M, Yoshimura N, Matsumura M, Yamamoto M, et al. Trabeculotomy ab externo: an alternative treatment in adult patients with primary open-angle glaucoma. Ophthalmic Surg. 1993;24(11):735–9.
4. Rosenquist R, Epstein D, Melamed S, Johnson M, Grant WM. Outflow resistance of enucleated human eyes at two different perfusion pressures and different extents of trabeculotomy. Curr Eye Res. 1989;8(12):1233–40.
5. Seibold LK, Soohoo JR, Ammar DA, Kahook MY. Preclinical investigation of ab interno trabeculectomy using a novel dual-blade device. Am J Ophthalmol. 2013;155(3):524–9.e2.

6. Minckler D, Baerveldt G, Ramirez MA, Mosaed S, Wilson R, Shaarawy T, et al. Clinical results with the Trabectome, a novel surgical device for treatment of open-angle glaucoma. Trans Am Ophthalmol Soc. 2006;104:40–50. Pubmed Central PMCID: 1809927
7. Francis BA, See RF, Rao NA, Minckler DS, Baerveldt G. Ab interno trabeculectomy: development of a novel device (Trabectome) and surgery for open-angle glaucoma. J Glaucoma. 2006;15(1):68–73.
8. Mosaed S, Dustin L, Minckler DS. Comparative outcomes between newer and older surgeries for glaucoma. Trans Am Ophthalmol Soc. 2009;107:127–33. Pubmed Central PMCID: 2814584
9. Mansberger SL, Gordon MO, Jampel H, Bhorade A, Brandt JD, Wilson B, et al. Reduction in intraocular pressure after cataract extraction: the Ocular Hypertension Treatment Study. Ophthalmology. 2012;119(9):1826–31. Pubmed Central PMCID: 3426647
10. Ophthalmology AAo. Elevated Episcleral Venous Pressure. 2017. https://www.aao.org/bcscs-nippetdetail.aspx?id=52ea963b-4164-480a-880b-6a79ed3f4772.
11. Akil H, Chopra V, Huang AS, Swamy R, Francis BA. Short-term clinical results of ab interno trabeculotomy using the Trabectome with or without cataract surgery for open-angle glaucoma patients of high intraocular pressure. J Ophthalmol. 2017;2017:8248710. Pubmed Central PMCID: 5412169
12. Gonnermann J, Bertelmann E, Pahlitzsch M, Maier-Wenzel AB, Torun N, Klamann MK. Contralateral eye comparison study in MICS & MIGS: Trabectome(R) vs. iStent inject(R). Graefes Arch Clin Exp Ophthalmol. 2017;255(2):359–65.
13. Khan M, Saheb H, Neelakantan A, Fellman R, Vest Z, Harasymowycz P, et al. Efficacy and safety of combined cataract surgery with 2 trabecular microbypass stents versus ab interno trabeculotomy. J Cataract Refract Surg. 2015;41(8):1716–24.
14. Kurji K, Rudnisky CJ, Rayat JS, Arora S, Sandhu S, Damji KF, et al. Phaco-trabectome versus phaco-iStent in patients with open-angle glaucoma. Canad J Ophthalmol J. 2017;52(1):99–106.
15. Mizoguchi T, Nishigaki S, Sato T, Wakiyama H, Ogino N. Clinical results of Trabectome surgery for open-angle glaucoma. Clin Ophthalmol. 2015;9:1889–94. Pubmed Central PMCID: 4607056
16. Akil H, Chopra V, Huang A, Loewen N, Noguchi J, Francis BA. Clinical results of ab interno trabeculotomy using the Trabectome in patients with pigmentary glaucoma compared to primary open angle glaucoma. Clin Exp Ophthalmol. 2016;44(7):563–9.
17. Shoji N, Kasahara M, Iijima A, Takahashi M, Tatsui S, Matsumura K, et al. Short-term evaluation of Trabectome surgery performed on Japanese patients with open-angle glaucoma. Jpn J Ophthalmol. 2016;60(3):156–65.
18. Bussel II, Kaplowitz K, Schuman JS, Loewen NA, Trabectome SG. Outcomes of ab interno trabeculectomy with the trabectome by degree of angle opening. Br J Ophthalmol. 2015;99(7):914–9. Pubmed Central PMCID: 4501175
19. Lee JW, Yick DW, Tsang S, Yuen CY, Lai JS. Efficacy and safety of Trabectome surgery in Chinese open-angle glaucoma. Medicine. 2016;95(15):e3212. Pubmed Central PMCID: 4839803
20. Hardik A, Parikh PR, Dhaliwal A, Kaplowitz KB, Loewen NA. Trabectome patient selection, preparation, technique, management, and outcomes. touch Ophthalmol. 2015;8(2):5. Epub 2015
21. Hu K, Gazzard G, Bunce C, Wormald R. Ab interno trabecular bypass surgery with Trabectome for open angle glaucoma. Cochrane Database Syst Rev. 2016;15(8):CD011693.
22. Minckler DS, Baerveldt G, Alfaro MR, Francis BA. Clinical results with the Trabectome for treatment of open-angle glaucoma. Ophthalmology. 2005;112(6):962–7.
23. Mosaed S. The first decade of global trabectome outcomes. touch Ophthalmol. 2014;8(2):113–9.
24. Jea SY, Francis BA, Vakili G, Filippopoulos T, Rhee DJ. Ab interno trabeculectomy versus trabeculectomy for open-angle glaucoma. Ophthalmology. 2012;119(1):36–42.
25. Okeke CO, Miller-Ellis E, Rojas M, Trabectome Study G. Trabectome success factors. Medicine. 2017;96(24):e7061. Pubmed Central PMCID: 5478308

26. Pahlitzsch M, Davids AM, Zorn M, Torun N, Winterhalter S, Maier AB, et al. Three-year results of ab interno trabeculectomy (Trabectome): Berlin study group. Graefes Arch Clin Exp Ophthalmol. 2018;256:611–9.
27. Ahuja Y, Pyi SMK, Malihi M, Hodge DO, Sit AJ. Clinical results of ab interno trabeculotomy using the trabectome for open-angle glaucoma: the Mayo clinic series in Rochester, Minnesota. Am J Ophthalmol. 2013;156:97.
28. Neiweem AE, Bussel II, Schuman JS, Brown EN, Loewen NA. Glaucoma surgery calculator: limited additive effect of phacoemulsification on intraocular pressure in ab interno trabeculectomy. PLoS One. 2016;11(4):e0153585. Pubmed Central PMCID: 4831696
29. Kaplowitz K, Bussel II, Honkanen R, Schuman JS, Loewen NA. Review and meta-analysis of ab-interno trabeculectomy outcomes. Br J Ophthalmol. 2016;100(5):594–600.
30. Lavia C, Dallorto L, Maule M, Ceccarelli M, Fea AM. Minimally-invasive glaucoma surgeries (MIGS) for open angle glaucoma: a systematic review and meta-analysis. PLoS One. 2017;12(8):e0183142. Pubmed Central PMCID: 5574616
31. Roy P, Loewen RT, Dang Y, Parikh HA, Bussel II, Loewen NA. Stratification of phaco-trabectome surgery results using a glaucoma severity index in a retrospective analysis. BMC Ophthalmol. 2017;17(1):30. Pubmed Central PMCID: 5360039
32. Vold SD, Dustin L, Trabectome Study G. Impact of laser trabeculoplasty on Trabectome(R) outcomes. Ophthalmic Surg Lasers Imaging. 2010;41(4):443–51.
33. Klamann MK, Gonnermann J, Maier AK, Bertelmann E, Joussen AM, Torun N. Influence of Selective Laser Trabeculoplasty (SLT) on combined clear cornea phacoemulsification and Trabectome outcomes. Graefes Arch Clin Exp Ophthalmol. 2014;252(4):627–31.
34. Dang Y, Kaplowitz K, Parikh HA, Roy P, Loewen RT, Francis BA, et al. Steroid-induced glaucoma treated with trabecular ablation in a matched comparison with primary open-angle glaucoma. Clin Exp Ophthalmol. 2016;44(9):783–8.
35. Ngai P, Kim G, Chak G, Lin K, Maeda M, Mosaed S. Outcome of primary trabeculotomy ab interno (Trabectome) surgery in patients with steroid-induced glaucoma. Medicine. 2016;95(50):e5383. Pubmed Central PMCID: 5268022
36. Anton A, Heinzelmann S, Ness T, Lubke J, Neuburger M, Jordan JF, et al. Trabeculectomy ab interno with the Trabectome(R) as a therapeutic option for uveitic secondary glaucoma. Graefes Arch Clin Exp Ophthalmol. 2015;253(11):1973–8.
37. Ting JL, Damji KF, Stiles MC, Trabectome Study G. Ab interno trabeculectomy: outcomes in exfoliation versus primary open-angle glaucoma. J Cataract Refract Surg. 2012;38(2):315–23.
38. Bussel II, Kaplowitz K, Schuman JS, Loewen NA, Trabectome Study G. Outcomes of ab interno trabeculectomy with the trabectome after failed trabeculectomy. Br J Ophthalmol. 2015;99(2):258–62. Pubmed Central PMCID: 4316927
39. Fellman RL, Feuer WJ, Grover DS. Episcleral venous fluid wave correlates with Trabectome outcomes: intraoperative evaluation of the trabecular outflow pathway. Ophthalmology. 2015;122(12):2385–91. e1
40. Minckler D, Mosaed S, Dustin L, Ms BF, Trabectome Study G. Trabectome (trabeculectomy-internal approach): additional experience and extended follow-up. Trans Am Ophthalmol Soc. 2008;106:149–59. discussion 59–60. Pubmed Central PMCID: 2646453
41. Jordan JF, Wecker T, van Oterendorp C, Anton A, Reinhard T, Boehringer D, et al. Trabectome surgery for primary and secondary open angle glaucomas. Graefes Arch Clin Ex Ophthalmol. 2013;251(12):2753–60. Pubmed Central PMCID: 3889259
42. Francis BA, Minckler D, Dustin L, Kawji S, Yeh J, Sit A, et al. Combined cataract extraction and trabeculotomy by the internal approach for coexisting cataract and open-angle glaucoma: initial results. J Cataract Refract Surg. 2008 Jul;34(7):1096–103.
43. Berk TA, An JA, Ahmed IIK. Inadvertent cyclodialysis cleft and hypotony following ab-interno trabeculotomy using the Trabectome device requiring surgical repair. J Glaucoma. 2017;26(8):742–6.
44. Osman EA, AlMobarak F. Ciliochoroidal effusion with persistent hypotony after trabectome surgery. Indian J Ophthalmol. 2015;63(3):272–4. Pubmed Central PMCID: 4448246

45. Maeda M, Watanabe M, Ichikawa K. Evaluation of trabectome in open-angle glaucoma. J Glaucoma. 2013;22(3):205–8.
46. Kaplowitz K, Schuman JS, Loewen NA. Techniques and outcomes of minimally invasive trabecular ablation and bypass surgery. Br J Ophthalmol. 2014;98(5):579–85. Pubmed Central PMCID: 4108346
47. Jea SY, Mosaed S, Vold SD, Rhee DJ. Effect of a failed trabectome on subsequent trabeculectomy. J Glaucoma. 2012;21(2):71–5.
48. Töteberg-Harms M, Rhee DJ. Limited success of selective laser trabeculoplasty following failed combined phacoemulsification cataract extraction and *ab interno* trabeculectomy (Trabectome). Am J Ophthalmol. 2013;156:936–40. Aug 7 Epub ahead of print
49. Grover DS, Godfrey DG, Smith O, Shi W, Feuer WJ, Fellman RL. Outcomes of Gonioscopy-assisted Transluminal Trabeculotomy (GATT) in eyes with prior incisional glaucoma surgery. J Glaucoma. 2017;26(1):41–5.
50. Grover DS, Godfrey DG, Smith O, Feuer WJ, Montes de Oca I, Fellman RL. Gonioscopy-assisted transluminal trabeculotomy, ab interno trabeculotomy: technique report and preliminary results. Ophthalmology. 2014;121(4):855–61.

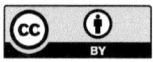

Hydrus Microstent

5

Panagiotis Laspas and Norbert Pfeiffer

5.1 Introduction

The Hydrus Microstent (Ivantis Inc., Irvine, CA, USA) is an intracanalicular scaffold which reduces the intraocular pressure (IOP) in order to treat glaucoma. The Microstent comes preloaded in a delivery system designed for *ab-interno* implantation under gonioscopic visualization. This is performed through the trabecular meshwork into Schlemm's canal typically in conjunction with planned cataract surgery. The implantation procedure is relatively intuitive and, if combined with cataract surgery, is usually performed at the end of surgery through the same corneal incision [1].

5.2 Material/Design

The Hydrus Microstent has a length of 8 mm. A 7-mm scaffold segment resides within the lumen of Schlemm's canal and a 1-mm inlet portion resides within the anterior chamber (Fig. 5.1) [1]. The Microstent is designed to fit the curvature of the canal without obstructing collector channel ostia located along the posterior wall (Fig. 5.2) [2]. The 8-mm Microstent is a modification of an earlier design that was 15 mm in length with a larger, nearly circular profile [3].

The Hydrus Microstent is made of nitinol (nickel–titanium alloy), a material with unique shape memory properties, which has been used widely in vascular medicine and other medical applications [4, 5]. The biocompatibility of nitinol for ocular applications has been reported previously and the Hydrus Microstent was initially evaluated in rabbit and primate ocular models [6, 7].

P. Laspas (✉) · N. Pfeiffer
Department of Ophthalmology, University Medical Center, Johannes Gutenberg University Mainz, Mainz, Germany
e-mail: Panagiotis.Laspas@unimedizin-mainz.de

© The Author(s) 2021
C. C. A. Sng, K. Barton (eds.), *Minimally Invasive Glaucoma Surgery*,
https://doi.org/10.1007/978-981-15-5632-6_5

Fig. 5.1 After
implantation into the
Schlemm's canal, the
Hydrus® Microstent is
visible through slit lamp
gonioscopic examination.
About 7 mm of the
Microstent lies in
Schlemm's canal,
scaffolding and dilating it.
A smaller segment of the
Microstent (about 1 mm)
prolapses at the site of
implantation through the
trabecular meshwork back
in the anterior chamber.
(Copyright permission
granted by Elsevier Inc.
according to STM
Guidelines [1])

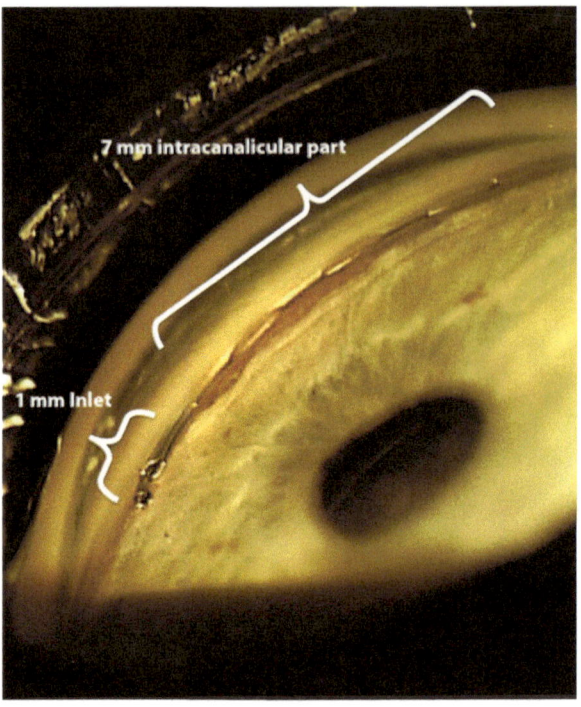

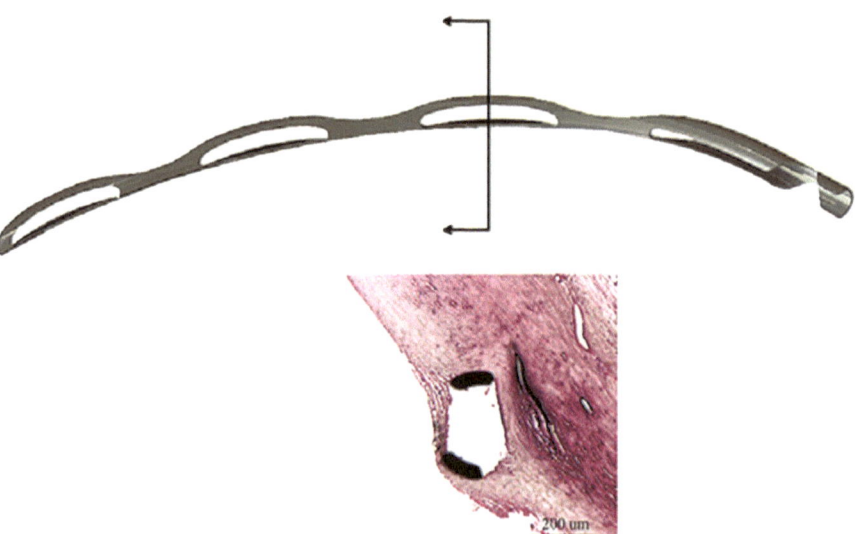

Fig. 5.2 The 8-mm Hydrus® Microstent consists of a scaffold of three windows and three spines
and an inlet region. The cross section of the Hydrus Microstent in the Schlemm's canal of a donor
eye shows the canal dilated, the trabecular meshwork stretched, and the access to collector channel
ostia free. (Copyright permission granted by Elsevier Inc. according to STM Guidelines [2])

5.2.1 Mechanism of Action

The Hydrus Microstent has a dual mode of action: First, this is a trabecular bypass minimally invasive glaucoma surgery (MIGS) device: the trabecular resistance, which plays a major role in the pathogenesis of open-angle glaucoma, is bypassed as aqueous gains direct access to the Schlemm's canal through the small inlet portion. Secondly, it dilates and scaffolds Schlemm's canal in order to increase the circumferential flow and maintain or facilitate access to collector channels (Fig. 5.3). Surgical procedures, such as canaloplasty, are based on a similar principle [8]. It has been hypothesized following ex vivo studies that elevated IOP itself may lead to alterations in the anatomy of trabecular meshwork and Schlemm's canal, which then becomes narrower or collapses [9]. The surgical dilation of Schlemm's canal leads to increased aqueous outflow and a reduction in IOP [10]. While canaloplasty offers a 360° dilation, the Hydrus Microstent can dilate only part of the canal's circumference. It creates a maximum Schlemm's canal dilation of 241 μm or approximately four to five times the natural cross-sectional area of the canal across its length [3].

A mathematical model has demonstrated that bypassing the trabecular meshwork increases the pressure and circumferential flow rate within Schlemm's canal, as well as the flow rate in collector channels adjacent to the bypass [11]. The same model showed that dilating Schlemm's canal adjacent to the bypass further reduces the pressure in the dilated region, which increases the circumferential flow rate even more. Thus, the Hydrus Microstent is unique in its design, which allows aqueous to flow without significant resistance from the anterior chamber directly into the collector channels. The small proximal 1-mm inlet of the Microstent in the anterior chamber bypasses the trabecular meshwork and permits a direct pathway for aqueous flow from the anterior chamber to Schlemm's canal, while the larger

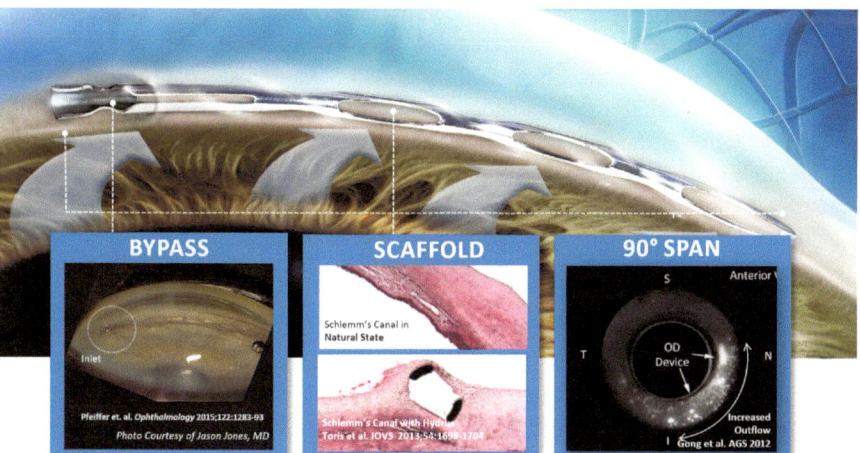

Fig. 5.3 The Hydrus® Microstent delivery system. (Copyright Ivantis Inc., Irvine, CA, USA; reproduced with permission)

intracanalicular portion provides persistent dilation of Schlemm's canal and access to the collector channel ostia.

5.3   Ex Vivo Testing

Grierson et al. reported the histological changes in primate and rabbit eyes after implantation of the Hydrus Microstent [7]. The host response to the Microstent within the ocular tissues at the anterior chamber angle was judged to be minimal: there was no evidence of tissue degeneration near the Microstent or elsewhere within the eyes. No histopathological signs of metallosis such as depigmentation, apoptosis, or tissue necrosis were present and there was no evidence of significant intraocular inflammation. A low-grade mononuclear immune response involving a few scattered macrophages was present in some tissues both close to and remote from the Microstent. An extremely thin capsule wall was found around the Microstent, consisting of one to two thin spindle-shaped fibroblasts without a substantial fibrous collagen component.

Johnstone et al. used scanning electron microscopy to assess the structure of the outer wall of Schlemm's canal after Microstent implantation in human cadaveric eyes [2]. Particulate debris was found at the site of the Microstent but did not occlude Schlemm's canal. Collector channels were regularly visible with intact margins and were not obstructed or compressed.

The mechanism of action of the device was tested in anterior segment perfusion models using human donor eyes [3, 12, 13]. Gulati et al. and Hays et al. performed experiments using the 8 mm version of the Microstent, while Camras et al. tested the effect of the previous 15 mm version. Overall, these studies confirmed an increase in outflow facility, compared with controls after sham treatment. This increase in outflow facility was more profound when the IOP was elevated. This implies that eyes with higher outflow resistance can be expected to have a greater improvement in outflow and therefore a greater decrease in IOP with the Hydrus Microstent. In addition, it is possible that the Microstent prevented Schlemm's canal from closure and collapse when the IOP was elevated, a phenomenon which has been shown in studies of the anatomy of the angle tissues in eyes with raised IOP [9, 14]. The dilation of Schlemm's canal by the Hydrus Microstent enabled the aqueous outflow to be measurably higher in eyes with significant IOP elevation, even though only one-quarter of the entire Schlemm's canal was stented. Another interesting finding in the study of Camras et al. [12] was that the improved outflow was attributable only to the presence of the Microstent itself and not by the implantation process or the subsequent histological changes in the trabecular meshwork or the Schlemm's canal: the outflow was not improved in eyes in which the Microstent was first implanted and then removed again. Histological examination of the site of implantation offered a possible explanation. It showed that the Schlemm's canal was widened by the Microstent, while the overlying trabecular meshwork appeared stretched but intact. Thus, damage to the angle structures by Hydrus Microstent implantation or the Microstent itself was very mild and was not likely to reduce trabecular resistance.

Fig. 5.4 The trimodal mechanism of action of the Hydrus® Microstent. (Copyright Ivantis Inc., Irvine, CA, USA; reproduced with permission)

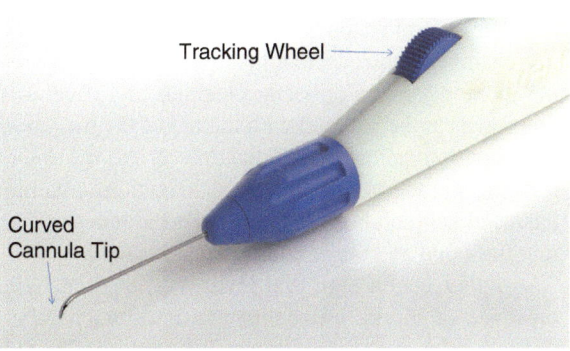

Tracking Wheel

Curved Cannula Tip

5.4 Surgical Technique

The Hydrus Microstent comes preloaded in a sterile delivery cannula (Fig. 5.4). The cannula is slightly curved so as to conform to the morphology of the angle and the Schlemm's canal. During implantation, the Hydrus Microstent is fed along 3 clock hours of Schlemm's canal. In order to facilitate this, the cannula can be rotated on the injector, permitting the surgeon to optimize his or her hand orientation for implantation. The device is inserted into the anterior chamber through a small clear-corneal paracentesis. Visualization of the angle via a goniolens is required for the precise implantation of the Hydrus Microstent. The cannula penetrates the trabecular meshwork at a very small angle almost tangential to its surface, so as to cannulate Schlemm's canal. Subsequently, the tracking wheel on the delivery system is used to slowly advance and implant the Hydrus Microstent, while keeping the cannula tip firmly in place. When approximately 1 mm of the proximal Microstent protrudes as an inlet from the trabecular meshwork into the anterior chamber, the delivery system is fully released.

5.5 Site of Implantation

The most common site for the implantation of the Hydrus Microstent is the nasal quadrant due to its accessibility through a clear corneal temporal incision [15]. The nasal angle also has the highest concentration of collector channels [16]. However, bypassing the trabecular meshwork may not be sufficient for lowering the IOP in some eyes, as the distal conventional aqueous outflow pathway, such as the collector channels and aqueous veins, may be obstructed and may also confer significant resistance to aqueous outflow. Correct identification of the parts of the angle with functional collector channels and targeted implantation of the Hydrus Microstent could theoretically improve the efficacy of the stent in lowering IOP.

The intraoperative signs which indicate the success of *ab-interno* trabeculotomy can also be used to assess whether the Hydrus Microstent has been implanted correctly [17]. For example, the presence of an episcleral venous fluid wave (blanching of the episcleral venous plexus when balanced salt solution is injected into the anterior chamber) indicates that the trabecular bypass procedure is successful in accessing the downstream collector channels and aqueous veins. Fellman suggested that this wave can be induced with the aid of the irrigation and aspiration system: insert the irrigation and aspiration handpiece into the anterior chamber with the infusion turned off, then initiate maximal irrigation, creating a high-pressure gradient for balanced salt solution to surge from the anterior chamber through the Microstent into the canal and the venous collector system.

Another useful sign that Hydrus Microstent implantation is successful is the presence of blood reflux into the anterior chamber from the Microstent lumen under low-pressure conditions. When the IOP is lower than the pressure in the episcleral veins, retrograde blood flow through patent collector channels and Schlemm's canal can occur. Implantation of the Hydrus Microstent into Schlemm's canal further allows blood to flow from the Schlemm's canal into the anterior chamber. Grieshaber et al. showed that the postoperative IOP correlated with the quantity of blood reflux into Schlemm's canal in 28 eyes of African patients who underwent *ab-externo* canaloplasty [18]. In the same study, the patency of the collector channels was also checked by injecting fluorescein dye into Schlemm's canal using a flexible microcatheter. However, this technique required conjunctival peritomy, which would defeat the objective of the *ab-interno* approach and compromise the success of subsequent glaucoma filtration surgery if indicated. *Ab-interno* procedures for assessing the conventional outflow system spare the conjunctiva and can provide valuable information regarding Hydrus Microstent placement and the likelihood of success for Schlemm's canal surgery. For example, Saheb et al. injected dye through the inlet of the Microstent after implantation in order to assess the anatomy and patency of the distal outflow pathway [15]. Furthermore, high-resolution imaging of the conventional outflow system can also help to determine the optimal site of implantation. Kagemann et al. used spectral domain ocular coherence tomography (OCT) to noninvasively assess Schlemm's canal, collector channels, and the intrascleral venous plexus [19, 20]. Further evolution of the imaging techniques and the introduction of OCT angiography may aid in planning optimal Hydrus Microstent placement and for predicting its probability of success.

5.6   Patients

Suitable patients for Hydrus Microstent implantation are those with primary open-angle glaucoma and pseudoexfoliative glaucoma. Contraindications include angle-closure glaucoma and secondary glaucoma, such as neovascular, uveitic, traumatic, steroid-induced, and lens-induced glaucoma. Furthermore, patients who previously underwent argon laser trabeculoplasty, cyclo-destructive procedures, trabeculectomy, tube shunt implantation, or any incisional glaucoma surgical procedure are not ideal candidates for Hydrus Microstent implantation: possible changes in the Schlemm's canal after such interventions can make implantation challenging or impossible. Hence, the surgical outcomes of Hydrus Microstent implantation in such patients remain uncertain [1].

5.7 Efficacy

The performance of the Hydrus Microstent in reducing IOP was evaluated in the HYDRUS II study: a prospective, single-masked, randomized controlled clinical trial conducted in seven European centers [1]. Patients were randomized to either cataract surgery combined with Hydrus Microstent implantation or cataract surgery alone and then followed up for 2 years. In order to accurately determine the efficacy of the surgery, patients underwent a washout of their hypotensive medications, similar to the protocol in the Ocular Hypertension Treatment Study [21] (Table 5.1).

One year after Hydrus Microstent implantation in combination with cataract surgery, the mean washed-out IOP decreased significantly by 9.7 mmHg (from 26.3 mmHg to 16.6 mmHg) compared with preoperative IOP. This effect persisted for 2 years after surgery, with the mean washed out diurnal IOP only 0.3 mmHg higher than that at 1 year at 16.9 mmHg. There was also a significant decrease in IOP at 1 year for eyes which underwent cataract surgery alone, with a mean reduction of 9.2 mmHg (from 26.6 mmHg to 17.4 mmHg). However, at 2 years, there was an increase in IOP to 19.2 mmHg in eyes which underwent cataract surgery alone, and this was significantly higher than the 2-year IOP in eyes which underwent Hydrus Microstent implantation in combination with cataract surgery.

Combined Hydrus Microstent implantation and cataract surgery were also associated with a reduction in glaucoma medications, with 77.1% and 72.3% of patients requiring no medications to achieve target IOP at 1 year and 2 years after surgery, respectively. Amongst patients who underwent cataract surgery alone, the proportion of patients who were medication-free at 1 year and 2 years after surgery was significantly lower compared with those who underwent combined Hydrus Microstent implantation and cataract surgery, at 49% and 36.4%, respectively. Moreover, patients who underwent combined Hydrus Microstent implantation and

Table 5.1 The efficacy of Hydrus® Microstent either as a standalone procedure or in combination with cataract surgery as reported in a number of studies [1, 8, 15, 22–24]

Group	Procedure	Follow-up	Pre-OP IOP	Post-OP IOP
Pfeiffer et al. [1]	Hydrus + Cataract Surgery	2 years	26.3 mmHg*	16.9 mmHg*
Ahmed et al. [15]	Hydrus + Cataract Surgery	6 months	17.9 mmHg	15.3 mmHg
Fea et al. [22]	Hydrus + Cataract Surgery	2 years	19.4 mmHg	15.7 mmHg
Al-Mugheiry et al. [23]	Hydrus	2 years	18.1 mmHg	15.3 mmHg
Fea et al. [24]	Hydrus	1 years	23.1 mmHg	16.5 mmHg
Gandolfi et al. [8]	Hydrus	2 years	24.0 mmHg	15.0 mmHg

*In the study by Pfeiffer et al., washout of glaucoma medication was performed in order to accurately determine the efficacy of Hydrus® Microstent implantation

cataract surgery required only half the mean number of glaucoma medications at 2 years compared with those who underwent cataract surgery alone.

The results of the Hydrus II study are similar to that of other smaller case series. Ahmed et al. reported the 6-month outcomes of 28 eyes with mild-to-moderate primary open-angle glaucoma after combined phacoemulsification and Hydrus implantation [15]. Baseline IOP was 17.9 ± 4.1 mmHg with 2.4 ± 1.0 glaucoma medications, and washed-out IOP was 29.9 ± 5.8 mmHg before surgery. The IOP and the mean number of glaucoma medications at 6 months were significantly reduced to 15.3 ± 2.3 mmHg and 0.1 ± 0.4, respectively. Fea et al. reported the 2-year results of 92 eyes that underwent combined cataract surgery and Hydrus Microstent implantation [22]. This was a retrospective study with no washout of glaucoma medications. Nevertheless, a 20% reduction in the mean IOP from 19.4 mmHg preoperatively to 15.7 mmHg at 2 years after surgery was observed. In a single-center and single-surgeon observational study, Al-Mugheiry et al. reported the 2-year results of 25 eyes which underwent combined Hydrus Microstent implantation and cataract surgery. At the end of 2 years, the mean medicated IOP was reduced from 18.1 (±3.6) mmHg to 15.3 (±2.2) mmHg [23].

The HORIZON study was a 24-month prospective, multicenter, single-masked randomized controlled trial which compared the reduction in IOP and medication use in subjects who underwent combined cataract surgery and Hydrus Microstent implantation (HMS, $n = 369$) with those who underwent cataract surgery alone (NMS, $n = 187$). At 24 months, 77.3% of the HMS group eyes achieved ≥20% reduction in unmedicated modified diurnal IOP (MDIOP) compared with 57.8% of NMS group eyes (difference = 19.5%, 95% confidence interval [CI] 11.2%–27.8%, $p < 0.001$). The mean ± standard deviation decrease in unmedicated MDIOP was −7.6 ± 4.1 mmHg in the HMS group and −5.3 ± 3.9 mmHg in the NMS group at 24 months (difference = 2.3 mmHg, 95% CI −3.0 to −1.6, $p < 0.001$). The safety profile was similar in both groups with no serious ocular adverse events related to the microstent [24]. These results confirmed the findings of the HYDRUS II study, that the efficacy of combined phacoemulsification and Hydrus Microstent implantation in lowering the IOP and glaucoma medications was superior to phacoemulsification alone.

Although Hydrus Microstent implantation is typically performed in combination with cataract surgery, the device can also be implanted as a solo procedure. Fea et al. reported the 1-year outcomes of Hydrus Microstent implantation as a solo procedure in 31 eyes (20 phakic, 11 pseudophakic) with primary open-angle glaucoma [25]. One year after surgery, the mean IOP decreased by 6.6 ± 5.6 mmHg (from 23.1 mmHg to 16.5 mmHg) and 47% of eyes were medication-free. This nonrandomized prospective study also compared the results of Microstent implantation with selective laser trabeculoplasty. At 1 year, IOP reduction was similar between Hydrus Microstent implantation and selective laser trabeculoplasty. However, eyes that underwent Hydrus Microstent implantation required significantly fewer medications to achieve target IOP compared with those which underwent selective laser trabeculoplasty, even though the eyes which underwent Hydrus Microstent implantation had more severe glaucoma. Gandolfi et al. reported the

2-year results of stand-alone Hydrus Microstent implantation compared with canaloplasty [8]. There was a significant and similar IOP decrease in both groups, from 24 ± 6 mmHg to 15 ± 3 mmHg in eyes that underwent Hydrus Microstent implantation and from 26 ± 4 mmHg to 16 ± 2 mmHg in eyes which underwent canaloplasty. In the COMPARE study, Ahmed et al. randomized 152 eyes from 152 patients with open-angle glaucoma to standalone MIGS consisting of either one Hydrus Microstent or two iStent Trabecular Micro-Bypass devices in a prospective, multicenter, randomized clinical trial. At 12 months, the Hydrus group had a higher rate of complete success (39.7% vs. 13.3%, $p < 0.001$) and reduced medication use (difference = −0.6 medications, $p = 0.004$), with more patients in the Hydrus group being medication-free (difference = 22.6%, $p = 0.0057$) [26].

5.8 Safety

Hydrus Microstent implantation is associated with a favorable safety profile [24, 27]. In the Hydrus II and HORIZON studies, the visual acuity of eyes that underwent combined cataract surgery with Hydrus Microstent implantation was similar to that of eyes after cataract surgery alone [1, 24]. Adverse events, such as cornea punctate staining, erosion of the corneal epithelium, stromal edema, endothelial folds, anterior chamber cells, and flare, were generally mild. All these were observed in the early postoperative period, with resolution within 4 weeks. In the course of the follow-up in the Hydrus II study, the formation of peripheral anterior synechiae (Fig. 5.5) was observed in six eyes at 1 year and nine eyes at 2 years after Hydrus Microstent implantation. Serious ocular adverse events were rare and not attributed to the procedure in the opinion of the investigators (acute vitreomacular traction, anterior ischaemic optic neuropathy, retinal detachment, and macular edema) [1]. A study by Ahmed et al. reported a low incidence of corneal edema, hyphema, and peripheral anterior synechiae [15]. The presence of peripheral anterior synechiae was not related to an increase in IOP in the HORIZON study [24].

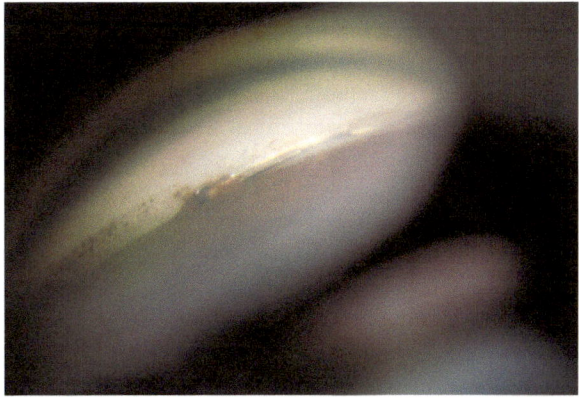

Fig. 5.5 Gonioscopy photograph showing peripheral anterior synechiae formation at the inlet of the Hydrus® Microstent. (Copyright Chelvin Sng, FRCSEd; reproduced with permission)

In a retrospective study by Fea et al., which included 92 eyes with combined Hydrus Microstent implantation and cataract surgery, one patient developed hyphema exceeding 2.0 mm in the early postoperative period and this resolved spontaneously without any sequelae [25]. The placement of the Hydrus Microstent was not satisfactory in two eyes and intraoperative repositioning was performed. Peripheral anterior synechiae without Microstent obstruction was observed in eight eyes, and iris occlusion of the device inlet occurred in one eye, which was treated with argon laser 8 months after the surgery. In one eye, the Microstent was malpositioned (outside Schlemm's canal) and the IOP was above target. This patient subsequently required trabeculectomy at 18 months. Al-Mugheiry et al. reported the outcomes of Hydrus Microstent implantation in 25 eyes by a surgeon with no prior surgical experience with the Microstent [23]. Despite the surgical inexperience, there were very few intraoperative complications. Hyphema occurred in two eyes during Microstent insertion. In one eye, the Microstent could not be fully inserted at the first attempt, but it was successfully inserted in another position at the second attempt. The postoperative adverse events on day 1 were mild-to-moderate anterior uveitis (12 eyes), mild corneal edema (7 eyes), micro-hyphema (7 eyes), or hyphema >1.5 mm (2 eyes). In one eye with microhyphema, there was an associated IOP spike (28 mmHg) and in one eye with a 2-mm hyphema, there was a blood clot seen at the opening of the Microstent, but this resolved spontaneously after a week. There was no correlation between day 1 complications and outcome.

Stand-alone Hydrus Microstent implantation was also found to be safe for phakic eyes, with a low incidence of adverse events being reported. In the prospective study by Fea et al., IOP spikes occurred in 2 out of 31 eyes (6.45%) on the first postoperative day [25]. After temporary treatment with systemic acetazolamide, the IOP was normalized in all eyes by the third postoperative day. There was a transient decrease in visual acuity in three eyes (9.68%) on the first postoperative day, which was due to corneal edema secondary to an IOP spike in one eye and hyphema in two eyes. Visual acuity returned to baseline by 1 week after the surgery in all three cases. Gandolfi et al. reported that hyphema was the most common post-operative adverse event (4 out of 21 eyes) [8]. The hyphema cleared completely over a few days in all cases. An early postoperative IOP spike (≥ 30 mmHg within the first 48 h) occurred in one eye after Hydrus Microstent implantation. Peripheral anterior synechiae developed in four eyes during follow-up, which was treated with a YAG laser procedure. Ahmed et al. reported that there was no significant difference in adverse events at one year between study eyes which underwent standalone Hydrus Microstent implantation compared with those which underwent implantation of two iStent Trabecular Micro-Bypass devices in the COMPARE study. Two subjects in the two iStent group required subsequent glaucoma surgery due to uncontrolled IOP despite maximum medical therapy, while none of the subjects in the Hydrus group required additional incisional glaucoma surgery. Ocular adverse events in both groups were mostly mild and transient [26].

In summary, Hydrus Microstent implantation may be associated with transient IOP spikes, hyphema, stent malposition or obstruction and the development of peripheral anterior synechiae. IOP spikes occur mostly in the early postoperative period and can be easily managed with glaucoma medications. Bleeding in the anterior chamber can vary from a circulating or micro-hyphema to a large hyphema. This is typically transient and self-resolving within a few days or weeks. Microstent malposition is associated with impaired stent function and surgical intervention may be required in these cases. Development of peripheral anterior synechiae is relatively common postoperatively, but is without clinical significance in most of the cases. However, synechial formation at the Hydrus Microstent inlet can result in stent obstruction, and this may be relieved by laser treatment in some cases. Clinically significant and long-standing hypotony or other potentially sight-threatening complications have not been described so far with Hydrus Microstent implantation, as its capacity to reduce IOP is limited by episcleral venous pressure.

5.9   Conclusion

Hydrus Microstent implantation in combination with cataract surgery or as a solo procedure is safe and effective for the treatment of primary open-angle glaucoma. This Schlemm's canal scaffold lowers IOP to the mid-teens and reduces glaucoma medication use for up to 2 years. Hence, it is promising as a long-term treatment modality for patients with mild to moderate primary open-angle glaucoma.

References

1. Pfeiffer N, et al. A randomized trial of a Schlemm's canal microstent with phacoemulsification for reducing intraocular pressure in open-angle glaucoma. Ophthalmology. 2015;122(7):1283–93.
2. Johnstone MA, et al. Effects of a Schlemm canal scaffold on collector channel ostia in human anterior segments. Exp Eye Res. 2014;119:70–6.
3. Gulati V, et al. A novel 8-mm Schlemm's canal scaffold reduces outflow resistance in a human anterior segment perfusion model. Invest Ophthalmol Vis Sci. 2013;54(3):1698–704.
4. Beeley NR, et al. Development, implantation, in vivo elution, and retrieval of a biocompatible, sustained release subretinal drug delivery system. J Biomed Mater Res A. 2006;76(4):690–8.
5. Ko GY, et al. Obstruction of the lacrimal system: treatment with a covered, retrievable, expandable nitinol stent versus a lacrimal polyurethane stent. Radiology. 2003;227(1):270–6.
6. Olson JL, Velez-Montoya R, Erlanger M. Ocular biocompatibility of nitinol intraocular clips. Invest Ophthalmol Vis Sci. 2012;53(1):354–60.
7. Grierson I, et al. A novel Schlemm's canal scaffold: histologic observations. J Glaucoma. 2015;24(6):460–8.

8. Gandolfi SA, et al. Comparison of surgical outcomes between canaloplasty and Schlemm's canal scaffold at 24 Months' follow-up. J Ophthalmol. 2016;2016:3410469.
9. Johnstone MA, Grant WG. Pressure-dependent changes in structures of the aqueous outflow system of human and monkey eyes. Am J Ophthalmol. 1973;75(3):365–83.
10. Johnstone MA, Grant WM. Microsurgery of Schlemm's canal and the human aqueous outflow system. Am J Ophthalmol. 1973;76(6):906–17.
11. Yuan F, et al. Mathematical modeling of outflow facility increase with trabecular meshwork bypass and Schlemm Canal dilation. J Glaucoma. 2016;25(4):355–64.
12. Camras LJ, et al. A novel Schlemm's canal scaffold increases outflow facility in a human anterior segment perfusion model. Invest Ophthalmol Vis Sci. 2012;53(10):6115–21.
13. Hays CL, et al. Improvement in outflow facility by two novel microinvasive glaucoma surgery implants. Invest Ophthalmol Vis Sci. 2014;55(3):1893–900.
14. Moses RA, et al. Schlemm's canal: the effect of intraocular pressure. Invest Ophthalmol Vis Sci. 1981;20(1):61–8.
15. Saheb H, Ahmed II. Micro-invasive glaucoma surgery: current perspectives and future directions. Curr Opin Ophthalmol. 2012;23(2):96–104.
16. Bill A. Some aspects of aqueous humour drainage. Eye (Lond). 1993;7(Pt 1):14–9.
17. Fellman RL, Grover DS. Episcleral venous fluid wave: intraoperative evidence for patency of the conventional outflow system. J Glaucoma. 2014;23(6):347–50.
18. Grieshaber MC, et al. Clinical evaluation of the aqueous outflow system in primary open-angle glaucoma for canaloplasty. Invest Ophthalmol Vis Sci. 2010;51(3):1498–504.
19. Kagemann L, et al. Identification and assessment of Schlemm's canal by spectral-domain optical coherence tomography. Invest Ophthalmol Vis Sci. 2010;51(8):4054–9.
20. Kagemann L, et al. 3D visualization of aqueous humor outflow structures in-situ in humans. Exp Eye Res. 2011;93(3):308–15.
21. Mansberger SL, et al. Reduction in intraocular pressure after cataract extraction: the ocular hypertension treatment study. Ophthalmology. 2012;119(9):1826–31.
22. Fea AM, Rekas M, Au L. Evaluation of a Schlemm canal scaffold Microstent combined with phacoemulsification in routine clinical practice: two-year multicenter study. J Cataract Refract Surg. 2017;43(7):886–91.
23. Al-Mugheiry TS, et al. Microinvasive glaucoma stent (MIGS) surgery with concomitant phakoemulsification cataract extraction: outcomes and the learning curve. J Glaucoma. 2017;26(7):646–51.
24. Samuelson TW, Chang DF, Marquis R, et al. A Schlemm canal microstent for intraocular pressure reduction in primary open-angle glaucoma and cataract: the HORIZON study. Ophthalmology. 2019;126:29–37.
25. Fea AM, et al. Hydrus Microstent compared to selective laser trabeculoplasty in primary open angle glaucoma: one year results. Clin Exp Ophthalmol. 2017;45(2):120–7.
26. Ahmed IIK, Fea A, Au L, et al. A prospective randomized trial comparing Hydrus and iStent microinvasive glaucoma surgery implants for standalone treatment of open-angle glaucoma: the COMPARE study. Ophthalmology. 2020;127:52–61.
27. Yook E, Vinod K, Panarelli JF. Complications of micro-invasive glaucoma surgery. Curr Opin Ophthalmol. 2018;29:147–54.

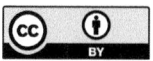

XEN Gel Implant

Leon Au and Ingeborg Stalmans

6.1   Device Design and Evolution

The concept of the XEN Glaucoma Treatment System was initially developed at the Lions Eye Institute in Perth, Australia. It was commercialized by the company AqueSys, Inc. (Fort Worth, Texas, USA) which later was acquired by Allergan plc (Dublin, Ireland) in 2015. The concept was to create a subconjunctival aqueous drainage pathway similar to trabeculectomy, but via an *ab-interno* approach. The XEN Gel Implant is a 6-mm hydrophilic collagen cylindrical implant comprising of cross-linked porcine gelatin. It has an external diameter of 150 μm and an internal lumen of 45 μm. It aims to provide a direct permanent communication between the anterior chamber and the subconjunctival space (Fig. 6.1). It is rigid when dry, but softens and swells externally after immersion in aqueous. The soft gelatinous property was thought to improve biocompatibility in the subconjunctival space and reduce the risk of erosion, while the small amount of external expansion aids device anchorage and minimizes migration. The XEN Glaucoma Treatment System received the CE mark in 2013 and was approved by the FDA in 2016. The lumen size of the XEN Gel Implant has changed from the initial 140 μm and later, 63 μm diameter versions, to the current, commercially available, 45 μm (also known as the XEN-45 implant), which is claimed to provide approximately 6–8 mmHg internal pressure resistance according to the Hagen–Poiseuille law and protect against post-operative hypotony [1].

L. Au (✉)
Manchester Royal Eye Hospital, Manchester University Foundation Trust, Manchester, UK

Medical Academic Health Sciences Centre, University of Manchester, Manchester, UK

I. Stalmans
Department of Ophthalmology, University Hospitals Leuven, Leuven, Belgium

Department of Neurosciences, Research Group of Ophthalmology, KU Leuven, Leuven, Belgium

© The Author(s) 2021
C. C. A. Sng, K. Barton (eds.), *Minimally Invasive Glaucoma Surgery*,
https://doi.org/10.1007/978-981-15-5632-6_6

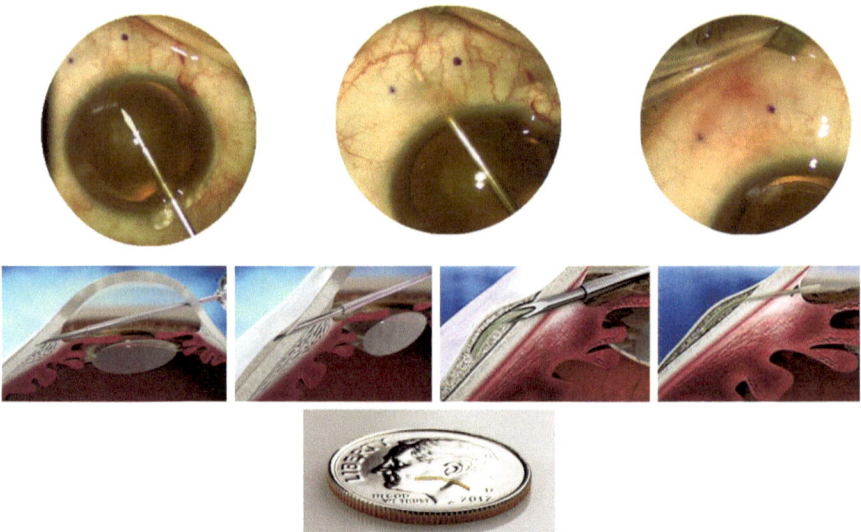

Fig. 6.1 The XEN Glaucoma Treatment System. (Copyright Allergan plc, Dublin, Ireland; reproduced with permission)

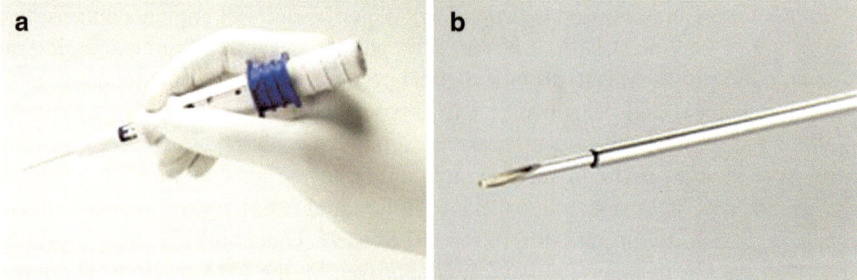

Fig. 6.2 The XEN Injector. (**a**) The XEN Gel Implant is preloaded in a disposable single-use injector. When the blue slider is moved forward, the XEN Gel Implant is injected into the subconjunctival space. (**b**) The tip of the injector comprises of a 27-gauge double beveled needle. (Copyright Allergan plc, Dublin, Ireland; reproduced with permission)

The XEN Gel Implant is preloaded in the XEN injector that is sterile and for single use only (Fig. 6.2). The injector comprises a straight 27-gauge double beveled needle with the XEN Gel Implant preloaded, a white surgical handle and a blue slider that deploys the implant. The injector advances across the anterior chamber through an inferotemporal clear corneal incision and delivers the XEN Gel Implant into the superonasal quadrant of the subconjunctival or sub-Tenon's space (Fig. 6.3). On completion of the deployment, the XEN Gel Implant should be placed 1 mm in the anterior chamber and 2 mm within the sclera, leaving a 3-mm extraocular portion under the conjunctiva. The implant should exit the sclera 3-mm posterior to the limbus, ideally creating a posterior filtration bleb. This is augmented by the use of

Fig. 6.3 Supero-nasal XEN Gel Implant associated with a diffuse bleb. (Copyright Leon Au, FRCOphth; reproduced with permission)

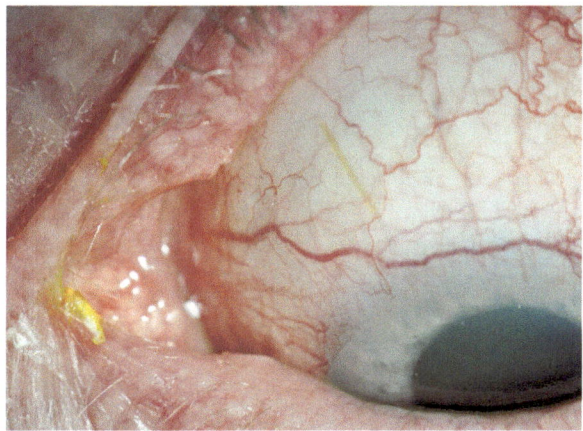

the antimetabolite, Mitomycin-C (MMC), which is typically given as a subconjunctival injection prior to device implantation.

6.2   Patient Selection

According to the CE mark, the XEN Gel Implant is intended to reduce intraocular pressure (IOP) in patients with primary open-angle glaucoma where previous medical treatments have failed. The Xen Glaucoma Treatment System was approved in the United States for the management of refractory glaucoma, where previous surgical treatment has failed, or in patients with primary open-angle glaucoma, pseudo-exfoliative or pigmentary glaucoma that is unresponsive to maximum tolerated medical therapy.

This procedure is suitable for patients with an open drainage angle, typically Shaffer grade 3 or above. The main advantages of the XEN Gel Implant over other filtering procedures include its less invasive surgical procedure which does not require conjunctival peritomy, the favorable safety profile, fast visual recovery, and short surgical duration, rendering this implant especially appropriate for patients who are unable to tolerate long surgical procedures or those who cannot accept prolonged visual recovery. Although designed as a stand-alone procedure, XEN implantation can be combined with phacoemulsification in patients with concurrent cataract. Since the implant is placed in the superonasal quadrant, other surgical options involving the supero-temporal quadrant are still an option in case of filtration failure.

The outcome after XEN implantation is dependent on the formation and maintenance of a filtering bleb. In contrast to conventional trabeculectomy where the outflow can be manipulated postoperatively via suture removal, the XEN Gel Implant is a fixed-flow device. As a result, its success is greatly dependent on the postoperative subconjunctival resistance. Therefore, patients at risk of bleb fibrosis are likely to have a less favorable surgical outcome, and careful patient selection is crucial for achieving success with this procedure. Known risk factors for fibrosis after filtering

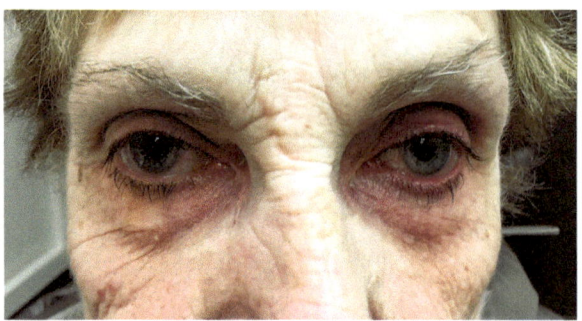

Fig. 6.4 A patient with deep and sunken superior sulcus which could result in difficulties in access during XEN surgery. (Copyright Ingeborg Stalmans, MD; reproduced with permission)

surgery include younger age, darker skin color, multiple topical glaucoma medications, diabetes, systemic autoimmune diseases, and a history of previous ocular surgery, especially procedures involving the conjunctiva. Moreover, preexisting intraocular and ocular surface inflammation increases the risk of postoperative fibrosis. Therefore, careful preoperative slit-lamp examination, including assessment of the inflammatory status, integrity, and mobility of the (superonasal) conjunctiva, as well as goniocopy to assess the angle, is mandatory for appropriate patient selection. Preoperative ocular surface disease and inflammation should be treated for ideally at least 1 month prior to surgery. Surgeons can consider altering or reducing the topical glaucoma medications before the surgery to reduce inflammation and decrease the preservative load, prescribing topical steroids or even switching from topical glaucoma medications to oral acetazolamide if there are no contraindications. Lid disease, blepharitis, and chronic dry eyes should be treated appropriately before the surgery.

It is important to achieve good surgical exposure for this procedure, especially because the procedure is performed with the eye in the primary position, as compared to conventional filtration surgery in which a corneal traction suture is used to rotate the eye downward. Hence patients need to be assessed preoperatively to ascertain whether the palpebral aperture is sufficiently wide and to identify factors which may cause surgical difficulties, including tight eyelids (e.g., history of contact dermatitis), a deep sunken sulcus or high cheekbones (Fig. 6.4). A comprehensive medical and surgical history should also be documented. Uncontrolled systemic hypertension or the use of oral anticoagulants for valvular heart disease increases the risk of intraocular and subconjunctival hemorrhage, the latter of which contributes to bleb fibrosis and surgical failure. Lastly, MMC is required for this procedure; hence, limbal stem cell failure and pregnancy are contraindications.

6.3   Surgical Technique

To indicate the intended implantation site, the conjunctiva is marked 3 mm from the limbus in the superonasal quadrant, close to the 12 o'clock position. Hydroexpansion of the tenon's capsule is performed by injecting MMC subconjunctivally in the target quadrant, at least 5 mm posterior to the limbus. An inferotemporal clear corneal incision is made at approximately 1 mm anterior to the limbus and an additional small incision is made nasally at the limbus. The anterior chamber is filled completely with a cohesive viscoelastic. The preloaded Xen injector is introduced across the anterior chamber through the main incision. The needle tip is aimed at the superonasal angle on the opposite side, ideally anterior to the pigmented trabecular meshwork and Schlemm's canal. Intraoperative gonioscopy can be used to position the injector needle precisely, before perforating the sclera to enter the subconjunctival space 2.5–3 mm behind the limbus. After ensuring that the entire bevel of the needle has exited the sclera and is within the subconjunctival space, the slider on the injector is moved forward. During the first half of the slider movement, the distal part of the implant is ejected from the needle tip into the subconjunctival space. Further movement of the slider forward results in the retraction of the needle into the injector while releasing the remainder of the implant in the sclera and anterior chamber. After the needle has fully retracted into the injector, it is removed from the anterior chamber. The position and the mobility of the subconjunctival segment of the implant are assessed and the correct length and position of the internal segment are confirmed by gonioscopy. Viscoelastic is removed from the anterior chamber and the incisions are hydrated (suturing is optional). The anterior chamber is irrigated and slightly pressurized to ensure that a filtration bleb is formed.

When XEN implantation is combined with phacoemulsification, cataract surgery is usually performed first. At the end of the cataract surgery, the anterior chamber is refilled with cohesive viscoelastic. XEN implantation can be performed through the main corneal incision used for phacoemulsification (if temporal) or an additional corneal incision can be made. The subsequent steps are similar to the solo procedure.

6.3.1   Avoiding Complications and Surgical Pearls

This section provides a step-by-step approach to the surgical procedure details, with practical recommendations on how to refine the surgical technique and to avoid and correct implant placement imperfections.

The surgeon can be seated superiorly or temporally. It is recommended that surgeons starting off with XEN implantation sit in their normal position for phacoemulsification, but also, as they gain confidence, try the alternative position. Similarly, there are several ways to hold the injector. The most comfortable hand position is also surgeon-dependent and is determined by a number of factors such as the hand size, the position of the surgeon relative to the patient, etc. However, holding the injector in the right hand when operating on a right eye and the left hand when operating on a left eye is advisable. Surgeons in training should try different seating and hand positions in the dry lab first, in order to find the most comfortable configuration. For the initial few cases, one should consider implanting pseudophakic patient with good surgical exposure and the right eye for the right-handed surgeon and vice versa. One should avoid implanting phakic patients until experienced with the technique.

The choice of anesthesia is also at the discretion of the surgeon. The majority of the procedures are performed under topical anesthesia, using anesthetic drops in combination with an intracameral supplement (separately injected in the anterior chamber or as a combo-product with the viscoelastic) and/or subconjunctival anesthesia (either in combination with the hydro-expansive fluid or separately). When used subconjunctivally, the anesthetic can be complemented with adrenaline as a vasoconstrictor. Some surgeons prefer a sub-tenon, peribulbar, or retrobulbar anesthesia. The advantage of the latter is deeper anesthesia, ensuring a painless procedure. In addition, for the novice, these provide akinesia, making the procedure easier. On the other hand, hydro-expansion may be more difficult because the patient cannot be instructed to look down to expose the posterior superior bulbar conjunctiva. We would encourage surgeons to move toward topical anesthesia when their techniques mature, because of the advantage of better access especially for hydro-expansion of the conjunctiva and delivery of MMC posteriorly into the fornix rather than at the limbus (Fig. 6.5).

To avoid excessive sub-conjunctival hemorrhage during hydro-expansion (which may obscure the implantation site and make the implantation procedure more challenging), a vasoconstrictor, such as topical apraclonidine (Iopidine®, Alcon, Fort Worth, Texas, USA) may be administered immediately prior to the surgery. This can counteract the hyperemia which is often caused by chronic glaucoma medication or pilocarpine administered preoperatively to constrict the pupil and protect the lens during standalone procedures. Alternatively, one can add adrenaline to the hydro-expansion fluid, as mentioned above or apply topical adrenaline. This has the potential disadvantage of pupil dilation, which can be prevented by preoperative topical pilocarpine. Ideally, one should use a fine (30G) needle for the hydro-expansion and carefully place the needle to avoid perforating conjunctival blood vessels. If sub-conjunctival hemorrhage does occur, one can immediately inject some fluid at the intended implantation site to prevent the blood from spreading to that area or compress the conjunctiva with a cotton tip and massage the blood away.

The use of antimetabolites in the hydro-expansion fluid is highly recommended. Although off-label, MMC is widely used in filtering surgery and accepted as common practice to prevent scarring and improve surgical outcomes. The concentration of the MMC can be titrated according to the patient profile which determines the anticipated scarring tendency (e.g., age, race, previous surgical history, etc.). The

Fig. 6.5 Posterior injection of mitomycin-C used for intra-tenon's hydroexpansion. (Copyright Ingeborg Stalmans, MD; reproduced with permission)

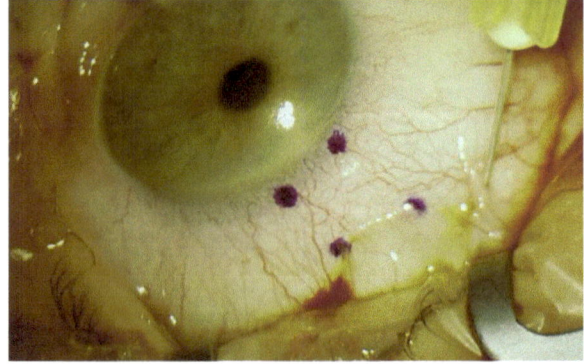

dose typically used is 0.02 mg in a volume of 0.1 mL, although it can vary between 0.01 and 0.05 mg. It is important to stress that the usage of MMC dosage greater than 0.02 mg is uncommon with the Xen and should be seen as exception rather than the rule, because of the higher risk of bleb avascularity and associated complications. To avoid an avascular bleb at the limbus and the risk of postoperative blebitis or endophthalmitis in rare cases [2, 3], MMC is injected as far posteriorly as possible and massaged backward with a cotton tip if it spreads close to the limbus.

After hydro-expansion, the fluid ideally lifts the conjunctiva slightly at the intended implantation site, to reduce the risk of conjunctival perforation with the injector needle as it comes out of the sclera, without obscuring the implantation site due to excessive chemosis.

The inferotemporal incision is made 1 mm from the limbus in order to approach the implantation site at the appropriate angle. In a patient with a prominent cheekbone, the surgeon may want to rotate the eye slightly between the injector and the side instrument, such that the injector is rotated away from the patient's cheek to a more temporal position. Alternatively, a more temporal incision may be considered, in combination with a more tangential approach to the superonasal angle rather than crossing the pupil axis (Fig. 6.6). A gentle face turn toward the temporal direction would also help to lower the cheekbone while the eye is brought slightly nasal to maintain a primary gaze during implantation. A nasal placement of the implant, however, is not recommended because of a higher incidence of dysesthesia from nasally placed blebs and potentially greater risk of implant erosion through the conjunctiva in nasally placed implants (presumably because of rubbing of the eyelid over the implant) (Fig. 6.7).

A cohesive viscoelastic material is used to fill the anterior chamber, providing a stable anterior chamber during implantation. This can also be removed more easily and more completely than a dispersive viscoelastic. We would recommend filling up the anterior chamber firmly during implantation, as it is more difficult to pierce

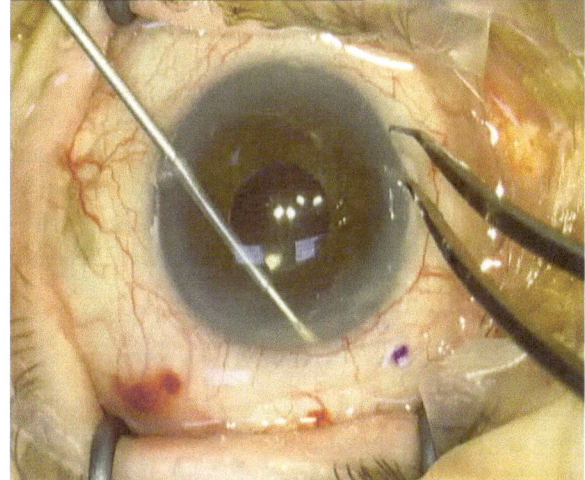

Fig. 6.6 Mild cyclo-rotation of the eye during XEN Gel Implant surgery, associated with a tangential approach of the injector which does not cross the pupil axis, so as to facilitate access to the superior-nasal quadrant of the eye in a patient with prominent cheekbones. (Copyright Leon Au, FRCOphth; reproduced with permission)

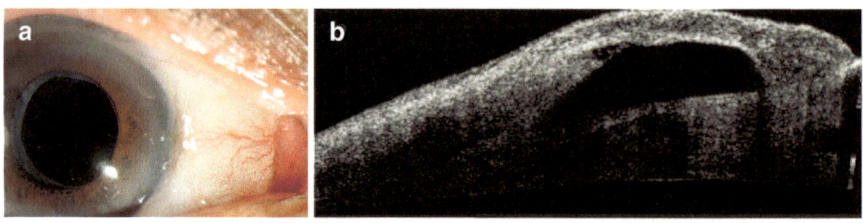

Fig. 6.7 Nasal placement of the XEN Gel Implant could result in a large nasal bleb. (**a**) A large nasal bleb which results in significant bleb dysesthesia. (**b**) Anterior segment optical coherence tomography image of the nasal bleb in (**a**), showing a large bleb cavity. (Copyright Chelvin Sng, FRCSEd; reproduced with permission)

sclera with the injector needle when the eye is soft. Similarly, avoid an excessively large corneal incision which allows viscoelastic to escape. The incision site needs to be marginally larger than 20 gauge to accommodate the injector. While small phaco wounds may be satisfactory, larger wounds can result in significant viscoelastic loss. A combined viscoelastic with anesthetic may also be used to complement the topical anesthesia and prevent pain during the procedure.

While entering the eye with the injector through the main port, small sidewise movements may facilitate smooth entry through the incision with the needle. A side instrument is used to stabilize the eye during the needle placement and injection. Various instruments can be used for this purpose, e.g., the Vera hook (Katena, USA), an iris spatula or a Bonn toothed forceps to grasp the cornea in the side point. As mentioned above, it is advisable to place the implant close to the 12 o'clock position, as nasal placement has been associated with bleb dysesthesia. Ideally, the implant is inserted between the pigmented trabeculum and Schwalbe's line. More posterior placement is associated with a higher risk of blood reflux from Schlemm's canal and ostium occlusion by the iris. More anterior placement can result in a very short intrascleral portion, instability of the implant and, occasionally, intracorneal placement. During the learning curve, it may be advisable to use an intraoperative indirect gonioscope to guide the injector needle while approaching the angle. However, with practice, the use of the gonioscope at this stage could later be omitted.

As the needle traverses the sclera, some forward pressure is required and the side instrument can serve to exert counterpressure. To reduce scleral resistance, and hence the amount of forward pressure on the injector required for placement, the injector can be gently rolled back and forth between the fingers creating a rotational movement of the needle. The needle should exit the sclera at 2.5–3 mm from the limbus. If necessary, the inserter can be tilted up- or downwards slightly during the insertion process to make the intrascleral portion longer or shorter. A longer intrascleral portion can reduce para-implant leakage and subsequent early hypotony, which may be more frequent in highly myopic eyes or those with thin sclera. A slow and controlled exit from the sclera is important to avoid puncturing the conjunctiva. There is a continuous debate about the ideal position of the implant in relation to the conjunctiva/tenon layers. Some surgeons prefer to aim the injector needle upwards, placing the implant in the superficial layers of the subconjunctival space, and increasing the chance of a freely mobile implant with easier drainage. In an ideal world, one would have the implant exit in the sub-Tenon's space behind Tenons insertion to avoid a thin bleb and implant erosion and maximize the use of the potential space available. The counterargument is that visualization of the patency of the XEN in the sub-Tenon's space is more difficult. Once the needle is fully advanced and the bevel has emerged completely from the sclera, the injector should be rotated 90° with the bevel facing the 12 o'clock position, before advancing the slider. During the first half of this manoeuver, the implant is ejected and during the second half, the needle is retracted. When the slider reaches the point of transition, a slight resistance can be felt in the finger moving the slider. At that point, one should pause, zoom out to get an overview of the cornea, and relax the hands to release any tension on either the injector or the side instrument. This is extremely important to avoid the so-called flicks, which are caused by tension on the injector during the retraction phase. At the point where the needle is retracted into the injector, the tip is released from the angle disengaging the anchorage. Any tension at that time can result in a flicking movement of the injector to one side or the other. This can drag the implant back into the anterior chamber causing an excessively long intraocular portion. The sudden movement can also result in a hemorrhage, an enlargement of the implantation canal or, in the case of a downward flick, iris trauma, and even cyclodialysis cleft formation in extreme cases.

When the injector is being retracted, the attention of the surgeon should therefore shift from the subconjunctival needle tip to the corneoscleral limbus. One should keep a forward bias on the injector to ensure constant contact between the injector and the angle. Only when the slider has reached the forward end of its travel (and therefore the needle is completely retracted), can the injector be removed safely from the anterior chamber. Premature removal can result in damage to the angle or dislocation of the implant. Common causes of suboptimal implant placement, most commonly implants that are too long in the anterior chamber, are incomplete needle advancement into the subconjunctival or sub-Tenon's space, incomplete slider advancement, early injector retraction, and flicks.

After implantation, it is important to check the position and mobility of the implant by gently moving the implant sidewise in both directions using a blunt instrument. Ideally, the implant should be 1 mm in the anterior chamber, 2 mm in the sclera, and 3 mm in the subconjunctival space (the so-called 1–2–3 configuration, see Fig. 6.8). The subconjunctival part of the implant should be straight and freely mobile sidewise. If the implant is not freely mobile or is curled, because it is stuck in Tenon's capsule (Fig. 6.9), the risk of occlusion by Tenon's, postoperative fibrosis and bleb failure is higher, even if the implant functions initially. Many surgeons will perform a primary needling in this situation. A 30G needle is inserted under the conjunctiva at a distance from the implant, and the tip of the implant is approached carefully avoiding the blood vessels. The Tenon's capsule is moved away from the implant by gently swiping over and under the implant with the needle, paying attention not to cut or pull out the implant. This maneuver should result in a straight and mobile implant. An alternative is to gently tease the implant using a pair of tying forceps. It is sometimes possible to free an implant from Tenon's by this method.

If no bleb is visible after removal of the viscoelastic, the internal position of the implant should be checked by performing gonioscopy. The ideal position of the

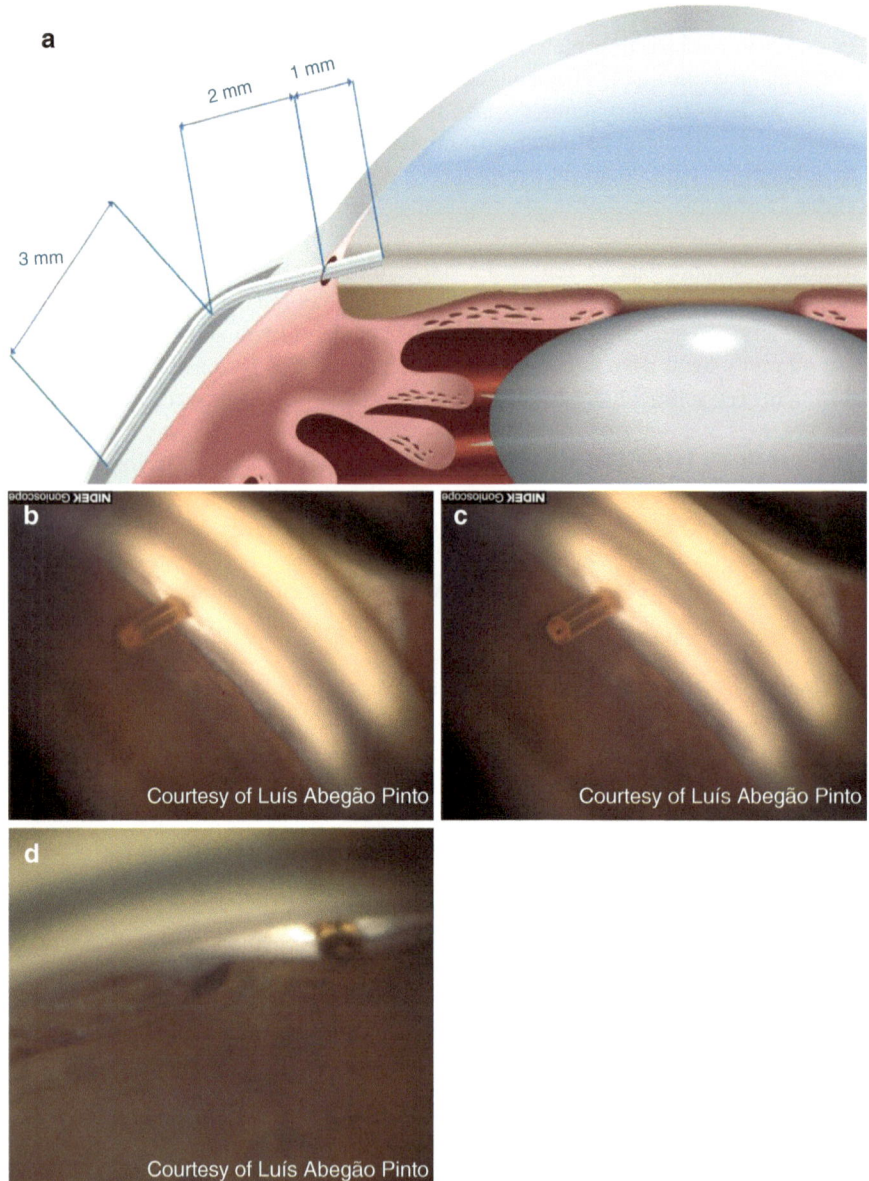

Fig. 6.8 The 1–2–3 configuration of the XEN Gel Implant. (**a**) The ideal placement of the XEN Gel Implant is 1 mm in the anterior chamber, 2 mm in the sclera, and 3 mm in the sub-conjunctival space. (Copyright Allergan plc, reproduced with permission) (**b**) Gonioscopic photograph focused on the entry site of the XEN Gel Implant, which is ideally between the pigmented trabeculum and the Schwalbe's line. (**c**) Gonioscopic photograph focused on the XEN Gel Implant which has an ideal intraocular segment of 1 mm. (**d**) Gonioscopic photograph showing a XEN Gel Implant which has an intraocular segment which is too short. (Copyright Luís Abegão Pinto, MD; reproduced with permission)

Fig. 6.9 A curled and immobile XEN Gel Implant which is impeded by Tenon's capsule. (Copyright Ingeborg Stalmans, MD; reproduced with permission)

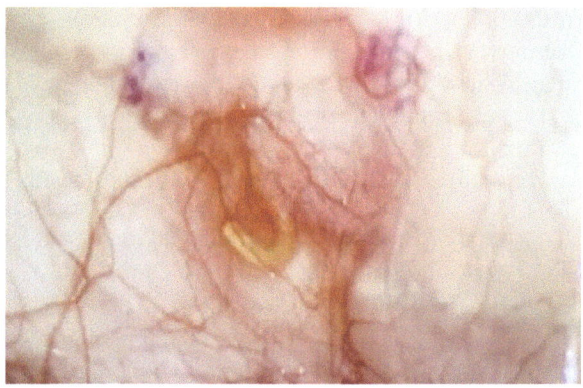

implant is between trabeculum and Schwalbe's line as mentioned previously. The iris is often pushed backward by the viscoelastic and the implant may appear free. However, if the implant is more posterior than the trabeculum, particularly if it is in contact with iris root at the scleral entry site, there is a risk of iris incarceration after viscoelastic washout. In which case, one might consider removing and reinserting the implant. An internal length of 0.5–1.5 mm, ideally 1 mm, is acceptable. If necessary, the length can be adjusted by gently grasping the extraocular portion of the implant through the conjunctiva with plain forceps and pushing it in or pulling it out. If the position of the implant is not satisfactory even after correction, removal, and reinsertion should be considered. To remove an implant, it may be convenient to first push the implant maximally into the anterior chamber using plain forceps e.g., Tying forceps. The implant can easily be removed from the anterior chamber using vitreoretinal forceps or aspirated using bimanual irrigation/aspiration. The injector needle is brought forward by moving the slider backward, the implant is placed in the needle again, and the insertion procedure is repeated. Care needs to be taken when handling the implant as it is now soft and can be fractured easily if excessive force is used. If there is any suspicion that the implant has been damaged, it would be more prudent to replace it with a new implant.

The final important point is the complete removal of the viscoelastic in the anterior chamber, which may otherwise block the implant in the early postoperative period and induce pressure spikes and meticulous hydration of the corneal incision. If the incisions are not watertight, they should be sutured. Thorough irrigation of the anterior chamber should result in a filtering bleb at the end of the surgery. If a filtering bleb is not visualized at the end of surgery, the implant and its position should be carefully examined and the procedure repeated if necessary. Intracameral antibiotics and subconjunctival steroids are recommended.

6.3.2   Postoperative Management

All pressure-lowering medications are discontinued immediately after the surgery. The typical postoperative regimen consists of a broad-spectrum topical antibiotic and intensive topical steroid (e.g., 2 hourly dexamethasone 0.1% or prednisolone acetate 1%). After 2 weeks, the antibiotic eyedrop can be discontinued while topical steroids can be gradually tapered over a course of 8–10 weeks. A longer duration of topical steroid may be required in eyes with significant or persistent conjunctival hyperemia or in pigmented eyes, which are at risk of more significant conjunctival scarring.

Typically, the IOP is low over the initial postoperative days. Based on the Hagen–Poiseuille's law and the dimensions of the XEN Gel Implant, the IOP should theoretically be 6–8 mmHg if the fluid passes solely through the implant without resistance in the subconjunctival space. In reality, day one IOP is often lower than 6 mmHg, presumably because the intrascleral canal produced by the injector is wider than the XEN Gel Implant, therefore allowing a small amount of para-tube leakage. In the days after the implantation, the outer diameter of the hydrophilic implant swells and its position in the sclera becomes tighter. Therefore the pressure after 1 week increases to typically around 10 mmHg.

Early hypotony usually resolves spontaneously in the first few postoperative days, requiring no additional treatment. If shallowing of the anterior chamber is a concern, a short-acting cycloplegic may be considered. Long-acting cycloplegics, such as atropine, are better avoided if the implant is posteriorly placed, because of the risk of obstructing the internal ostium of the implant with iris. In cases of significant anterior chamber shallowing or rarely when hypotony lasts 1–2 weeks after surgery, if accompanied by significant visual disturbance, corneal–lenticular touch, choroidal effusion, or maculopathy, slit-lamp injection of a small amount of dispersive visco-elastic can be used to temporize. Cohesive viscoelastics should be avoided as they may induce spikes in pressure.

A high IOP level on the first postoperative days is rare, assuming that the steps outlined above have been followed during the implantation procedure. A high-pressure spike is very suggestive of a mechanical cause. Gonioscopy should be performed to confirm correct implant placement and to rule out any mechanical blockage, e.g., by iris, blood, or fibrin. The most frequent cause of an early high-pressure spike is incomplete removal of the viscoelastic, in which case the pressure usually recovers in the first postoperative week. In cases of pronounced pressure spikes, anterior chamber washout should be considered. A limited hyphema generally resolves spontaneously, but if persistent or associated with an elevated pressure, a washout may rarely be required, ideally after a few days delay in order to reduce the risk of a rebleed.

If high pressure develops after the first postoperative week(s), again blockage of the internal ostium of the implant should be excluded gonioscopically. Other causes to be considered at this stage are a steroid response in combination with bleb encapsulation, especially if the bleb appears elevated. If the internal ostium is patent and there is no visible bleb elevation, then fibrosis around the implant is the more likely cause of the high pressure and needling or bleb revision may be considered. Needling is really only feasible if the implant is visible, revision can be carried out in either scenario. Encapsulation and fibrosis tend to develop after 3–4 postoperative weeks. If IOP elevation develops after 1–2 weeks, reversible mechanical obstruction of the XEN, with Tenon's rather actual fibrosis should be considered.

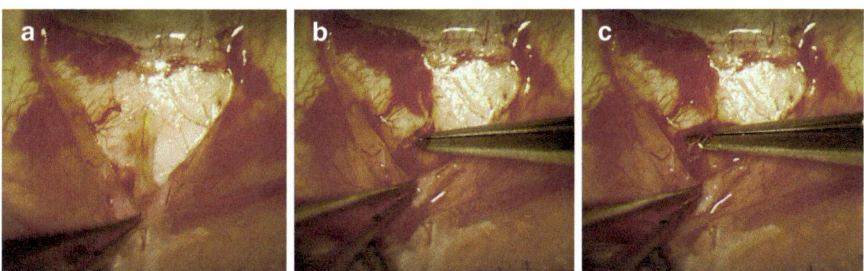

Fig. 6.10   XEN Gel Implant bleb revision. (**a**) A small fornix-based conjunctival peritomy is performed. (**b**) Subconjunctival fibrosis is carefully dissected off to expose and free up the XEN Gel
Implant. (**c**) Once the XEN Gel Implant is mobile and free, slow aqueous flow is visible from its
distal end. (Copyright Ingeborg Stalmans, MD; reproduced with permission)

Bleb revision is often performed under local anesthesia. A small fornix-based
conjunctival peritomy is performed and the subconjunctival fibrosis is carefully dissected off to expose the XEN implant. The implant is often wrapped in a "sock" of
tenon's tissue and a slow meticulous technique is required to free the implant without damaging it (Fig. 6.10). Once the XEN implant is mobile, one should be able to
detect a slow dripping of aqueous from its distal end. Visualization may be enhanced
using fluorescein drops and/or Vision Blue. If not, the implant itself might be
blocked and one should consider flushing the device using a lacrimal cannula on a
syringe containing BSS. If the device appears patent externally and internally but no
aqueous is seen egressing from the distal end, then a fresh device should be
implanted. Removal of the original non-functioning implant is unnecessary but is
easy to perform at the same time. If MMC is to be used during a revision, ideally it
should be applied after opening the conjunctiva but before freeing the XEN, in order
to avoid any chance of MMC reflux into the anterior chamber. After the revision is
complete, conjunctiva is closed in a similar fashion as conventional trabeculectomy.
The postoperative eyedrop regime is similar to standard XEN Gel Implant surgery.

6.4   Safety, Efficacy, and Clinical Results

The APEX study group reported the 2-year results of a multicenter, prospective,
nonrandomized open-label study of the XEN Gel Implant surgery in medically
uncontrolled open-angle glaucoma [4]. In 202 eyes with a mean preoperative medicated IOP of 21.4 ± 3.6 mmHg, the IOP was significantly reduced to 14.9 ± 4.5 mmHg
at 1 year and 15.2 ± 4.2 mmHg at 2 years (both $p < 0.001$). Medications were
reduced from 2.7 ± 0.9 preoperatively to 0.9 ± 1.1 at 1 year and 1.1 ± 1.2 at 2 years.
Overall, 51.1% and 47.7% of eyes were medication-free at 1 year and 2 years,
respectively. There was no difference in outcome between eyes which underwent
XEN implantation as a stand-alone procedure and those that underwent combined
phacoemulsification with XEN implantation. Success was defined as $\geq$20% IOP
reduction with the same or fewer glaucoma medications and 65.8% of eyes achieved

that at 2 years. These findings are consistent with other published retrospective and prospective studies reporting the outcome at 1 year [5–10] (Table 6.1).

In the US pivotal trial, Grover et al. reported the 12-month outcome of XEN surgery in refractory glaucoma where 84.6% of patients had a previously failed glaucoma procedure and 56.9% required ≥4 IOP lowering agents [10]. The average visual field mean deviation was −15.0 ± 7.7 dB and the mean cup-to-disk ratio was 0.82 ± 0.13. Despite the advanced nature of this group, 75.4% of patients achieved ≥20% IOP reduction with same or fewer medications at 12 months, resulting in a mean postoperative IOP of 15.9 ± 5.2 mmHg. Nine out of the 65 eyes (13.8%) did require a secondary glaucoma procedure during the 12 months period. It is worth noting that in this study, conjunctival peritomy was performed in all cases in order to apply the licensed MMC sponges (Mitosol, Mobius Therapeutics LLC, USA), which was different from our current implantation technique and could theoretically affect the outcome.

The postoperative needling rate of XEN surgery varies greatly. In the APEX study, the mean needling rate was 41.1% but it varied greatly between sites, ranging from 0% to ≥80% [4]. Over two-thirds of the needled eyes required only one episode and there was no difference between XEN alone and combined phaco-XEN surgeries. Similar needling rates were reported by others, supporting the importance of postoperative bleb management. [5–10]

The reported incidence of both intraoperative and postoperative complications was low. Numerical hypotony (IOP <6 mmHg) occurred in up to 20% of patients in the initial postoperative period but mostly resolved without interventions [4–10]. Other complications, including device obstruction by iris, conjunctival erosion resulting in implant exposure, endophthalmitis, and significant visual loss, were rare.

In a retrospective study, Schlenker and colleagues evaluated the outcome of XEN surgery versus trabeculectomy in uncontrolled glaucoma with no prior incisional surgery [11]. The results demonstrated no difference in efficacy, safety, and risk of failure between the two groups, with the XEN group favoring a quicker visual recovery but a higher needling rate.

Table 6.1 Summary of published XEN studies with 1-year follow-up

Authors	No. of cases	Surgery	Preop IOP mmHg	12mth IOP mmHg	≥20% IOP drop off Rx	Needling (%)
De Gregorio et al. [5]	41	Phaco-XEN	22.5 ± 3.7	13.1 ± 2.4	80.4% (IOP 6–17 no Rx)	2.4
Gala et al. [6]	13	XEN and phaco-XEN	16 ± 4	12 ± 3	41.7%	30.7
Hengerer et al. [7]	242	XEN and phaco-XEN	32.2 ± 9.1	14.2 ± 4.0	55.4%	27.7
Mansouri et al. [8]	149	XEN and phaco-XEN	20.0 ± 7.1	13.9 ± 4.3	57.7%	37
Tan et al. [9]	39	XEN	24.9 ± 7.8	14.5 ± 3.4	56.2% (IOP <18 no Rx)	51.3
Grover et al. [10]	65	XEN	25.1 ± 3.7	15.9 ± 5.2	75.4% (same or fewer Rx)	21

6.5   Off-Label Use

Although the XEN Gel Implant was licensed for use in open-angle glaucoma and refractory glaucoma uncontrolled with medications or prior glaucoma surgery, its filtering property resembles that of trabeculectomy hence could potentially be adopted in other subtypes of glaucoma. Sng and colleagues reported good efficacy with the XEN Gel Implant as a treatment for uncontrolled uveitic glaucoma [2]. In their cohort of 24 consecutive patients, XEN Gel Implant surgery achieved a remarkable 60.2% IOP reduction from a high baseline IOP of 30.5 ± 9.8 mmHg typically found in uveitic patients; 83.3% of patients avoided further surgery at 1 year. Nevertheless, caution should be exercised when considering the XEN Gel Implant for uveitic eyes due to the significantly higher risk of postoperative hypotony. In Sng's series, 20.8% of patients required anterior chamber reformation for hypotony. In addition, the implant could be occluded by inflammatory debris in uveitic eyes or by hypotonic/atrophic iris tissue if the position is too posterior. Angle closure is currently considered a contraindication for XEN implantation. In a case series of 19 angle-closure eyes, Sng et al. reported that combined XEN implantation with cataract surgery significantly reduced the IOP (11.7 ± 3.0 vs. 21.7 ± 3.7 mmHg, $p < 0.001$) and the number of glaucoma medications (0.2 ± 0.5 vs. 1.4 ± 0.7, $p < 0.001$) compared to baseline. The safety profile of XEN implantation in their small case series was similar to that reported for POAG eyes, though implant occlusion with iris occurred postoperatively in one angle closure eye [12]. However, they could not determine the additional effect of XEN implantation in lowering the IOP compared with phacoemulsification alone, and a randomized study comparing phacoemulsification alone with the combined procedure in angle-closure eyes is warranted. Successful XEN surgery has also been reported in patients with ICE syndrome and endothelial transplant as well as refractory glaucoma with previously failed trabeculectomy and two Ahmed valves [13, 14]. D'Alessandro and colleagues reported a novel combination of the XEN Gel Implant and the Baerveldt tube in the treatment of difficult refractory glaucoma [15]. It offers the potential advantage of immediate drainage of the XEN Gel Implant and the posterior diversion of aqueous over a large plate of Baerveldt implant. The smaller XEN implant in the anterior chamber is potentially more endothelial friendly than the larger glaucoma drainage implant. However, constant friction between the XEN Gel Implant and the much large Baerveldt tube may risk longer term implant fracture at this junction, thereby disconnecting the Baerveldt from the anterior chamber. There are also concerns that the XEN may slip out of the tube unless it is sutured securely, as the external diameter of the XEN is significantly less than the internal diameter of the Baerveldt. In addition, connecting the Baerveldt tube with the XEN Gel Implant does not necessarily prevent early postoperative hypotony, which can be a consequence of peri-implant aqueous flow [16]. Notably, most of these novel applications of XEN were performed in small numbers and their longer term results are yet to be determined.

6.6   Conclusion

The XEN Glaucoma Treatment System is currently the only procedure that targets the subconjunctival filtering space through an *ab-interno* approach. It offers a more significant reduction in IOP and medications than other *ab-interno* MIGS procedures. However, it is also arguably more technically demanding and a meticulous surgical approach is paramount. The creation of a filtering bleb requires careful pre- and postoperative management in order to secure success.

References

1. Vera VI, Horvath C. XEN gel stent: the solution designed by AqueSys. In: Samples JR, Ahmed IIK, editors. Surgical innovations in glaucoma. New York: Springer Science+Business Media; 2014. p. 189–98.
2. Sng CC, Wang J, Hau S, Htoon HM, Barton K. XEN-45 collagen implant for the treatment of uveitic glaucoma. Clin Exp Ophthalmol. 2018;46:339–45.
3. Kerr NM, Wang J, Sandhu A, Harasymowycz PJ, Barton K. Ab interno gel implant-associated bleb-related infection. Am J Ophthalmol. 2018;189:96–101.
4. Reitsamer H, Sng C, Vera V, Lenzhofer M, Barton K, Stalmans I, for the Apex study group. Two-year results of a multicenter study of the ab interno gelatin implant in medically uncontrolled open-angle glaucoma. Graefes Arch Clin Exp Ophthalmol. 2019;257:983–96.
5. De Gregorio A, Pedrotti E, Russo L, Morselli S. Minimally invasive combined glaucoma and cataract surgery: clinical results of the smallest ab interno gel stent. Int Ophthalmol. 2018;38:1129–34. https://doi.org/10.1007/s10792-017-0571-x.
6. Galal A, Bilgic A, Eltanamly R, Osman A. XEN glaucoma implant with mitomycin C 1-year follow-up: result and complications. J Ophthalmol. 2017;2017:5457246.
7. Hengerer FH, Kohnen T, Mueller M, Conrad-Hengerer I. Ab interno gel implant for the treatment of glaucoma patients with or without prior glaucoma surgery: 1-year results. J Glaucoma. 2017;26(12):1130–6.
8. Mansouri K, Guidotti J, Rao HL, et al. Prospective evaluation of standalone XEN gel implant and combined phacoemulsification-XEN Gel implant surgery: 1-year results. J Glaucoma. 2018;27(2):140–7.
9. Tan SZ, Walkden A, Au L. One-year result of XEN45 implant for glaucoma: efficacy, safety, and postoperative management. Eye. 2018;32(2):324–32.
10. Grover DS, Flynn WJ, Bashford KP, et al. Performance and safety of a new ab interno gelatin stent in refractory glaucoma at 12 months. Am J Ophthalmol. 2017;183:25–36.
11. Schlenker MB, Gulamhusein H, Conrad-Hengerer I, et al. Efficacy, safety, and risk factors for failure of standalone ab interno gelatin microstent implantation versus standalone trabeculectomy. Ophthalmology. 2017;124(11):1579–88.
12. Sng CCA, Chew PTK, Htoon HM, et al. Case series of combined XEN implantation and phacoemulsification in Chinese eyes: one-year outcomes. Adv Ther. 2019;36(12):3519–29.
13. Sandhu S, Dorey MW. Case report: Xen Ab Interno gel stent use in a refractory glaucoma patient with previous filtration surgeries. J Glaucoma. 2018;27(3):e59–60.
14. Hohberger B, Welge-Lüen UC, Lämmer R. ICE-syndrome: a case report of implantation of a microbypass Xen gel stent after DMEK transplantation. J Glaucoma. 2017;26(2):e103–4.
15. D'Alessandro E, Guidotti JM, Mansouri K, Mermoud A. XEN-augmented Baerveldt: a new surgical technique for refractory glaucoma. J Glaucoma. 2017;26(2):e90–2.
16. Sng CCA, Wang J, Barton K. Caution in using the XEN-augmented Baerveldt surgical technique. J Glaucoma. 2017;26:e257.

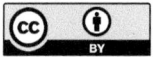

PRESERFLO MicroShunt

Nathan M. Kerr, Iqbal Ike K. Ahmed, Leonard Pinchuk, Omar Sadruddin, and Paul F. Palmberg

7.1   Introduction

Reducing intraocular pressure (IOP) remains the only proven treatment to prevent vision loss from glaucoma [1–3]. Under-treatment of glaucoma remains a significant issue and inadequate IOP reduction can increase the risk of vision loss [4]. Traditionally, trabeculectomy has been regarded as the gold standard in glaucoma surgery since it was described in the 1960s [5]. However, while one of the most effective IOP-lowering treatments, severe adverse events can occur, recovery can be prolonged and intense post-operative management is required.

N. M. Kerr (✉)
Centre for Eye Research Australia, Melbourne, VIC, Australia

Royal Victorian Eye and Ear Hospital, Melbourne, VIC, Australia
e-mail: nathan.kerr@eyeandear.org.au

I. I. K. Ahmed
Department of Ophthalmology and Vision Sciences, University of Toronto,
Toronto, ON, Canada

Prism Eye Institute, Mississauga, ON, Canada

L. Pinchuk
Ophthalmic Biophysics Center, Bascom Palmer Eye Institute, University of Miami Miller
School of Medicine, Miami, FL, USA

Santen Inc., Emeryville, CA, USA

O. Sadruddin
Santen Inc., Emeryville, CA, USA

P. F. Palmberg
Bascom Palmer Eye Institute, University of Miami Miller School of Medicine,
Miami, FL, USA

Anne Bates Leach Eye Hospital, Miami, FL, USA

© The Author(s) 2021   91
C. C. A. Sng, K. Barton (eds.), *Minimally Invasive Glaucoma Surgery*,
https://doi.org/10.1007/978-981-15-5632-6_7

Trabeculectomy is well-recognized to achieve significant and sustained reductions in IOP. In the tube versus trabeculectomy (TVT) study the mean IOP following trabeculectomy was 12.6 mmHg at 5 years. However, 37% of patients in this study developed complications in the early perioperative period and 18% required re-operation [6]. Furthermore, there is a significant surgical learning curve associated with trabeculectomy and a high level of surgical skill is required [7]. Intensive postoperative follow-up is mandatory to achieve optimum outcomes and perioperative interventions are frequent, with up to 78% of cases requiring some form of bleb manipulation and/or suture removal [8]. Although rare, sight-threatening complications following trabeculectomy can occur and include hypotony, choroidal effusions and suprachoroidal haemorrhage among others [6]. For these reasons, trabeculectomy is often reserved for late in the disease process when other treatments have failed [9].

The PRESERFLO® MicroShunt (Santen Pharmaceutical Co. Ltd., Osaka, Japan) is a new glaucoma drainage microtube that has been developed with the intention to provide significant and long-term IOP and glaucoma medication reduction similar to that of trabeculectomy but in a simpler, safer and less-invasive operation with faster recovery than conventional surgery. This chapter summarizes the development, lab testing, pre-clinical studies and human clinical trials for the MicroShunt.

7.2   Device Design and Development

There have been three major iterations in the design of the shunt to enhance ease of insertion, minimize complications and improve success rates. The final design, the PRESERFLO MicroShunt, is 8.5 mm long with an internal lumen of 70 μm and an outer diameter of 350 μm (Fig. 7.1). It received a CE mark in 2012. The length of the device was designed to achieve 1–2 mm in the anterior chamber, 3 mm within the sclera and 3 mm posterior to the needle tract wound. These dimensions summed to 8.5 mm in length. The lumen diameter was then approximated with the Hagen–Poiseuille equation to provide sufficient resistance to limit hypotony given published aqueous humour flow rates and viscosities [11]. The shunt is made of poly(styrene-*block*-isobutylene-*block*-styrene) or 'SIBS' material. The anterior end is bevelled to facilitate entry into the scleral tunnel and anterior chamber and is

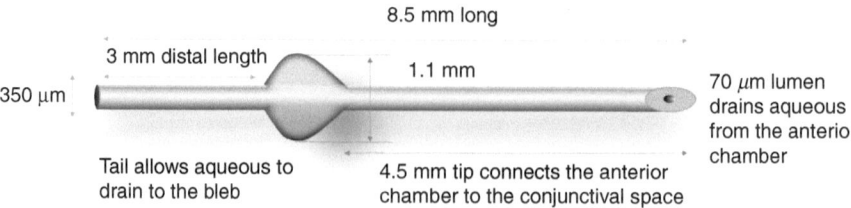

Fig. 7.1   PRESERFLO® MicroShunt. (Copyright Santen Pharmaceutical Co. Ltd., Osaka, Japan; reproduced with permission)

faced towards the cornea to enable visualization and clearing of the lumen if obstructed. Fixation fins are located approximately half-way down the shunt and serve three important functions. The fins fit snugly within the scleral tunnel and are designed to prevent leakage of aqueous around the tube, stop migration of the tube into the anterior chamber and orientate the shunt so that the bevel faces the cornea. The final design does not have a plate, reducing the complexity of insertion and minimizing the risk of diplopia.

The initial design, called the MIDI-Tube (an acronym for Miami InnFocus Drainage Implant), was trimmed in situ by the surgeon to approximately 11 mm long with an internal lumen of 70 μm and an outer diameter of 250 μm (Fig. 7.2). Early animal studies assessed the effect of lumen size on IOP lowering and found fewer complications and comparable IOP levels with a 70 μm lumen compared to larger 100 μm and 150 μm lumens [10]. A single fixation tab was located on one side to prevent migration into the anterior chamber and to enable insertion through a slotted needle with the fin protruding through the slot. The device was inserted through the scleral tunnel using this slotted needle inserter, however, due to the soft and flexible characteristics of the tube it would frequently jam in the inserter, and the surgeon would instead simply thread the MicroShunt through the scleral tunnel with forceps. The initial success rate, defined as an IOP ≤ 21 mmHg with a reduction from baseline of ≥20%, was low at 42% at 1 year in early human clinical trials [11]. However, it should be noted that in the first human trial (Bordeaux I), antimetabolites were not used and more than half of the patient population had failed previous glaucoma surgeries. In a subsequent clinical trial of 16 patients with previous failed incisional surgery (Bordeaux II), mitomycin-C (MMC) 0.2 mg/mL was applied for 2–3 min to only the sclera in the vicinity of the tube, and the success rate increased to 67% at 1 year [11].

A second-generation device, called the MIDI-Ray as it resembled a sting ray, was developed comprising a larger tube measuring 12 mm in length with an outer diameter of 350 μm, internal lumen of 100 μm connected to a plate 7 mm in diameter (Fig. 7.2) [11]. It was hypothesized that the plate would prevent encapsulation and eliminate the need for anti-metabolites [11]. However, the device had a high rate of hypotony due to the larger diameter tube and undesirable cystic bleb morphology. The MIDI-Ray did not enter large scale clinical trials.

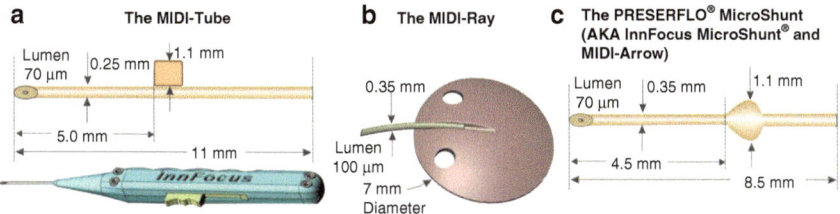

Fig. 7.2 The three major iterations in the design of the glaucoma shunt: (**a**) the MIDI-Tube; (**b**) the MIDI-Ray and (**c**) the PRESERFLO® MicroShunt, which is the final design. (Copyright Santen Pharmaceutical Co. Ltd., Osaka, Japan; reproduced with permission)

Fig. 7.3 Anterior
segment photograph
showing (**a**) the
PRESERFLO®
MicroShunt in the
anterior chamber and (**b**)
a diffuse bleb associated
with the PRESERFLO®
MicroShunt. (Copyright
Chelvin Sng, FRCSEd;
reproduced with
permission)

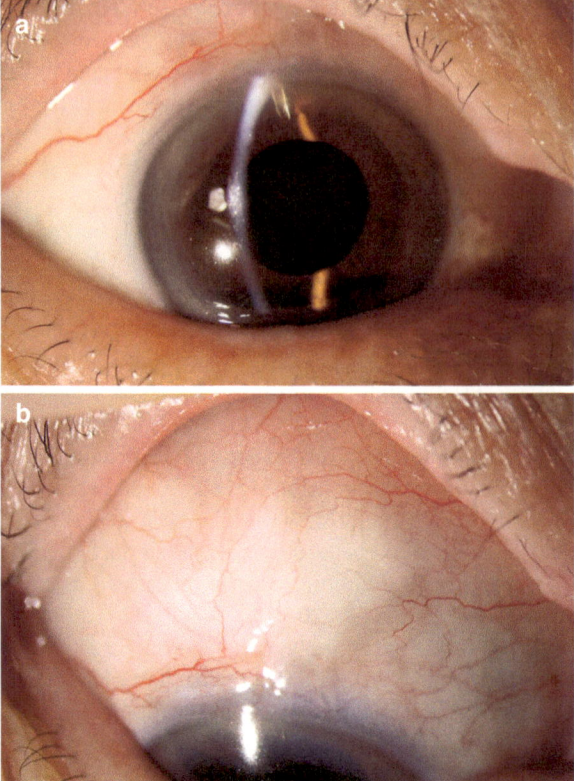

The third-generation device, called the MIDI-Arrow, comprised of symmetrical planar fins with a wingspan of 1.1 mm located midway along the length of an 8.5 mm SIBS tube with a 350 μm outer diameter and a 70 μm lumen. The MIDI-Arrow name was dropped due to concerns about patients believing an arrow would be placed in their eye. At that time, many of the implanting surgeons simply called the device the 'InnFocus device' or the 'InnFocus procedure', therefore the device was called the InnFocus MicroShunt®, often referred to as simply the 'IMS'. Santen Pharmaceutical Co. Ltd. acquired InnFocus Inc. in May 2016 and 3 years later renamed the device the PRESERFLO MicroShunt (Fig. 7.3).

7.3   Development of SIBS

Inflammation and fibrosis in the subconjunctival space may lead to surgical failure. Therefore, the selection of a biocompatible material that produces minimal inflammation is important to increase success. Traditional glaucoma drainage devices such as the Molteno (Molteno Ophthalmic Limited, Dunedin, New Zealand) or Baerveldt (Abbott Medical Optics, Santa Ana, CA) have been shown to elicit intense inflammatory reactions with multinucleated giant cells and the deposition of dense fibrous tissue surrounding the implants [12, 13].

Conventional implant materials such as polyether urethane slowly degrade in the body due to hydrolysis and oxidation [14]. This degradation attracts granulocytes (e.g. polymorphonuclear leukocytes) and macrophages leading to a foreign body reaction and capsule formation; features undesirable for a subconjunctival filtration device [15]. Silicones are more biostable than the polyurethanes but are often contaminated with unreacted starting materials as well as fillers and elicit a foreign body reaction [14]. The PRESERFLO MicroShunt is made of ultrapurified medical-grade poly(styrene-*block*-isobutylene-*block*-styrene) or SIBS, a novel biostable and biocompatible synthetic polymer devoid of cleavable group such as amides, esters, ureas, carbamates, etc. on both its backbone and side groups. First approved for medical use in 2004, SIBS has been widely used in cardiac stents due to its lack of biodegradation, absence of platelet activation, minimal tissue reaction and ability to be used as a drug-eluting system [16, 17].

Poly(styrene-*block*-isobutylene-*block*-styrene) is a synthetic polymer devoid of any sites prone to degradation by mechanisms such as oxidation, hydrolysis or enzymatic degradation (Fig. 7.4) [16]. Consisting of stable alternating secondary-and-quaternary carbons, SIBS is not prone to double bond formation that could lead to embrittlement or stress cracking [16]. Synthesized by cationic polymerization, SIBS can be injection and compression moulded and is stable under harsh conditions [18]. The SIBS material is soft and flexible and will conform to various shapes without surface cracking [19]. In addition, SIBS is a thermoformable material and will assume the shape it is placed in without a tendency to straighten as do the silicones tubes which are thermoset materials that tend to straighten over time. Silicones need to be secured in place, usually covered with a patch graft, in contrast to SIBS tubes which assume the shape of the globe. SIBS is sterilizable with ethylene oxide but not gamma-ray irradiation [19].

The biocompatibility of SIBS has been established in both animal and human studies. Discs of SIBS material were implanted in the cornea and sub-Tenon space

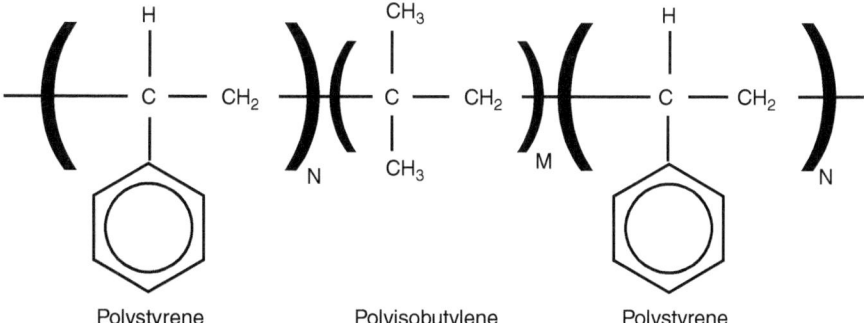

Fig. 7.4 Simplified structure of poly(styrene-block-isobutylene-block-styrene), or 'SIBS'. (Copy right Santen Pharmaceutical Co. Ltd., Osaka, Japan; reproduced with permission)

of normal rabbit eyes and compared against discs of silicone rubber [20]. The silicone discs showed angiogenesis, myofibroblasts and capsule formations, whereas there was no angiogenesis, myofibroblasts, nor intact capsules surrounding the SIBS material [20]. Further studies investigated the biocompatibility of a glaucoma drainage device made from SIBS in normal New Zealand white rabbits [21]. Glaucoma drainage devices made of SIBS were implanted into the anterior chamber while the distal tip was placed in the subconjunctival space [21]. Control animals underwent insertion of a similarly designed silicone tube [21]. At 3 months, haematoxylin–eosin staining revealed abundant collagen IV deposition around the silicone tubes with expression of alpha-smooth muscle actin [21]. In comparison, eyes implanted with the SIBS device showed a distinct absence of myofibroblasts, inflammatory cells and fibrosis [21]. In addition, encapsulation and neovascularisation were not observed in the SIBS group.

Glaucoma device patency was assessed by injection of fluorescein into the anterior chamber. All SIBS tubes remained patent out to 6 months while only two of the six silicone tubes were patent at 3 months [21].

7.4   Clinical Data

The safety and efficacy of the PRESERFLO MicroShunt have been evaluated in a number of clinical trials. In a multicentre, retrospective clinical trial, Beckers et al. reported the results of 91 patients with open-angle glaucoma who underwent either stand-alone MicroShunt insertion ($n = 73$) or combined cataract surgery and MicroShunt insertion ($n = 18$) [22]. All cases received MMC, but a varying concentration (0.2–0.4 mg/mL on sponges for 2–3 min). At 12 months, the mean IOP had reduced from a baseline of 24.3 mmHg on 2.4 medications to 13.3 mmHg on 0.4 medications with 83% of patients off all glaucoma medications [22]. The most common adverse event was transient numerical hypotony, occurring in 11% of patients [22]. All cases of hypotony resolved without intervention [22].

A second clinical trial examined the effect of MMC concentration on surgical outcomes [23]. In this retrospective two-centre study, patients with open-angle glaucoma were implanted with either the MicroShunt alone ($n = 66$) or in combination with cataract surgery ($n = 21$) [24]. Patients received either MMC 0.2 mg/mL near the limbus, MMC 0.4 mg/mL near the limbus or MMC 0.4 mg/mL deep in the subconjunctival conjunctival space [23]. For all patients, the duration of MMC exposure was 2–3 min. Overall there was a reduction in IOP and glaucoma medication requirements in all groups with the lowest IOP being in patients treated with MMC 0.4 mg/mL near the limbus [23]. In these patients, IOP reduced from a mean of 23.8 ± 5.3 mmHg on 2.4 ± 0.9 medications at baseline to 10.7 ± 2.8 mmHg on 0.3 ± 0.8 medications at 12 months [23]. There were no sight-threatening events in any group [23].

The patients who received MMC 0.4 mg/mL near the limbus were followed prospectively and the results presented at 2 and 3 years [16, 24]. All patients had primary open-angle glaucoma and had failed maximum tolerated medical therapy [16]. Patients with failed subconjunctival filtration surgery were excluded [16]. From a baseline IOP of 23.8 ± 5.3 mmHg on maximum tolerated medication therapy, 100% of patients achieved an IOP of 18 mmHg or lower at both 1 and 2 years [16]. The most common adverse events were mild and consisted of transient shallow anterior chamber and IOP < 5 mmHg (3/23, 13%) [16].

At 3 years, 100% of the patients continued to achieve an IOP ≤ 18 mmHg and 18 (82%) had an IOP of ≤14 mmHg [24]. The mean IOP at 3 years was 10.7 ± 3.5 mmHg, representing a 50% reduction in IOP [24]. Mean medication usage reduced from a baseline of 2.4 ± 0.9 medications to 0.7 ± 1.1 and 80% of patients were off glaucoma medications [24]. There were no sight-threatening complications and no patient lost >1 line of visual acuity [24]. The most common adverse events were transient hypotony (3/23, 13%) and transient choroidal effusions (2/23, 8.7%) [24]. All resolved spontaneously [24]. There were no cases of bleb leak, infection, tube exposure or persistent corneal oedema [24].

In August 2019, Santen Pharmaceutical announced the results of the US premarket approval (PMA), head-to-head study of the PRESERFLO MicroShunt versus trabeculectomy [25]. This prospective, randomized, controlled, single-masked, multicentre study compared standalone MicroShunt implantation with intraoperative 0.2 mg/mL MMC against stand-alone trabeculectomy with the same concentration of MMC. At 12 months, mean (± standard deviation) diurnal IOP was reduced from 21.1 ± 4.9 mmHg to 14.2 ± 4.4 mmHg in the MicroShunt group and from 21.1 ± 5.0 mmHg to 11.2 ± 4.2 mmHg in the trabeculectomy group. The mean number of glaucoma medications at month 12 was reduced in both groups, from 3.0 medications at baseline to 0.6 in the MicroShunt group and 0.3 in the trabeculectomy group, with 71.6% of subjects in the MicroShunt group being medication-free compared with 84.8% of subjects in the trabeculectomy group. Although the 12-month IOP was statistically lower in the trabeculectomy group compared with the MicroShunt group, trabeculectomy was associated with a greater incidence of hypotony at any time (51.1% vs. 30.6%), bleb leaks and lens opacity.

7.5 Patient Selection

The PRESERFLO MicroShunt is indicated for patients with open-angle glaucoma refractory to medical therapy. The MicroShunt can be performed alone or in combination with cataract surgery for patients with both refractory glaucoma and visually significant cataract. The MicroShunt provides a simple and fast alternative to primary trabeculectomy and eliminates the need for scleral flap dissection, iridectomy and post-operative suture lysis. Once efficacy and safety are fully established, the MicroShunt may allow for an earlier transition to surgical management. Because a significant proportion of patients are medication-free following the MicroShunt procedure compared to other MIGS procedures, it may be especially suited for patients with intolerance to topical glaucoma medications or adherence problems.

Due to its ability to achieve IOP in the low to mid-teens, the MicroShunt may be appropriate for patients with more advanced disease, unlike some other minimally invasive procedures. The MicroShunt can theoretically be placed in any quadrant, however as with trabeculectomy, prior failed subconjunctival filtration surgery may reduce surgical success rates. Inferior placement may increase the risk of bleb-related infection and is not recommended.

The PRESERFLO MicroShunt may be useful in the treatment of angle-closure glaucoma when combined with cataract surgery or in pseudophakic patients. Because the PRESERFLO MicroShunt shares features of both trabeculectomy and a glaucoma drainage device, it may potentially have a role in conditions such as iridocorneal endothelial cell syndrome, uveitic glaucoma and neovascular glaucoma. However, at the present time, there is limited data on the efficacy and safety of the device for these off-label indications.

7.6   Surgical Technique

The PRESERFLO MicroShunt comes in a sterile pre-packaged kit containing a 3 mm marking ruler, marking pen, sponges to apply MMC, a 1 × 1 mm triangular slit keratome knife to create a scleral pocket, and either a 25G or 27G needle.

The procedure is most commonly performed under a local anaesthetic block and the preferred site for implantation is superiorly at 11 or 1 o'clock (Fig. 7.5). Initially, a 6- to 8-mm wide peritomy is made at the limbus before Westcott scissors are used to dissect posteriorly for 8–10 mm, ensuring to dissect under Tenon's capsule. Bipolar diathermy is then used to achieve haemostasis before MMC application. Three sponges soaked in MMC, typically between 0.2 and 0.4 mg/mL, are placed under Tenon's for 3 min before irrigation with >20 mL of normal saline. Care should be taken to apply the sponges close to the limbus as well as deep in the flap. The

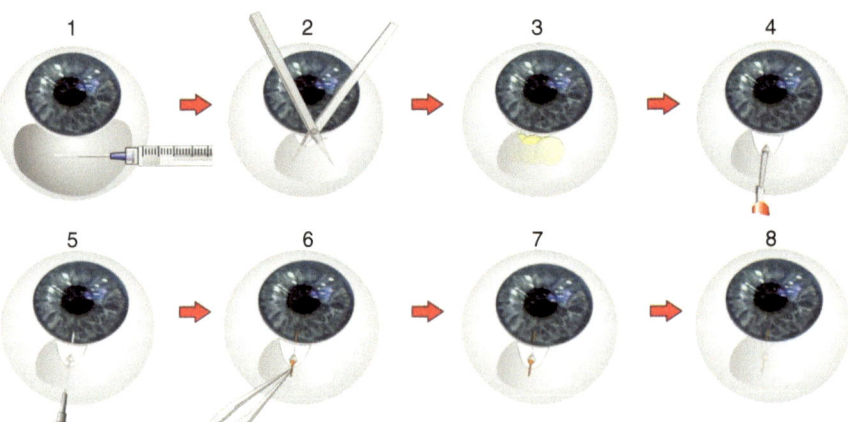

Fig. 7.5 PRESERFLO® MicroShunt implantation. (Copyright Santen Pharmaceutical Co. Ltd., Osaka, Japan; reproduced with permission)

ruler is used to mark 3 mm and a scleral tunnel fashioned with a slit keratome for 2 mm. A 25G needle is passed within the scleral tunnel to the apex before entering the anterior chamber in the plane of the iris and away from the corneal endothelium. The MicroShunt is inserted into the scleral tunnel with forceps and the wings secured within the tunnel (Fig. 7.6). The distal end is observed for flow (Fig. 7.7). If there is no flow, gentle pressure can be applied to the globe or the shunt can be flushed with a thin-walled 23G cannula if required. The distal end is tucked under Tenon's, which is advanced with the conjunctiva back to the limbus prior to conjunctival closure. The distal end should be checked to ensure it is not occluded with Tenon's and lastly it should be verified that there is no leak.

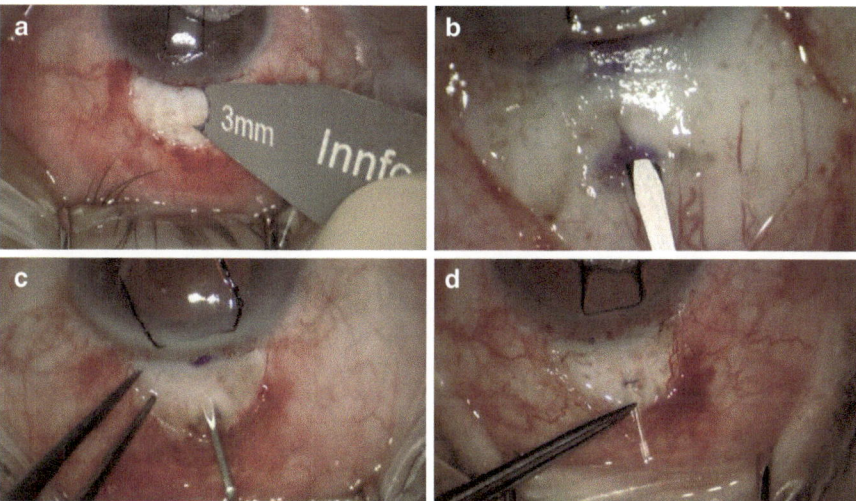

Fig. 7.6 Insertion of the PRESERFLO® MicroShunt. (**a**) A mark is made 3 mm from the surgical limbus. (**b**) A 2-mm shallow tunnel is formed in the sclera using a slit knife. (**c**) A 25-guage needle is passed through the tunnel to enter the anterior chamber. (**d**) The MicroShunt is inserted through the needle tract with the bevel up until the wedges are locked in the scleral incision. (Copyright Moorfields Eye Hospital and Keith Barton; reproduced with permission)

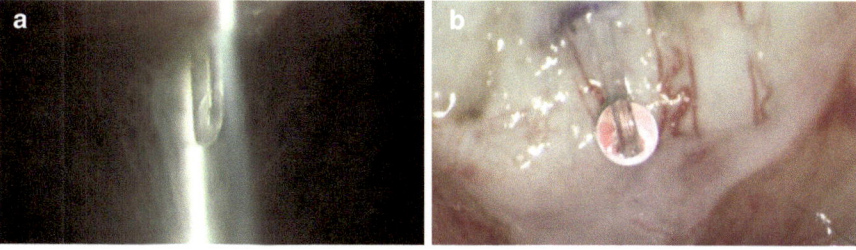

Fig. 7.7 The PRESERFLO® MicroShunt drains aqueous from the anterior chamber to the subconjunctival/subtenon space. (**a**) The proximal tip of the MicroShunt positioned in the anterior chamber. (**b**) Egress of aqueous from the distal end of the MicroShunt. (Copyright Moorfields Eye Hospital and Keith Barton; reproduced with permission)

7.7   Complications

7.7.1   Intraoperative Complications

Intraoperative complications are uncommon with the PRESERFLO MicroShunt. Potential complications include hyphaema or malposition of the shunt with occlusion by iris or placement of the tip of the device close to the endothelium with risk of endothelial cell damage. These are theoretical risks with any glaucoma drainage device inserted into the anterior chamber and can be avoided with careful surgical technique. Observation of the device directly through the cornea or with the aid of a goniolens can confirm safe placement of the device and in the event the surgeon is not pleased with the placement, the device can simply be pulled out of the scleral tunnel and repositioned in a new tunnel. Confirmation of flow through the device is indicative of no periannular leakage as well as non-obstruction of the tube lumen by iris or cornea.

7.7.2   Early Postoperative Complications

Extreme IOP fluctuations within the first week post-operatively with the MicroShunt are rare. Conventional drainage devices such as the Molteno or Baerveldt valves require tying off of the tube lumen to prevent hypotony as well as fenestration of the tube to allow some flow of aqueous humour to maintain the bleb. Similarly, trabeculectomy requires suture tension on the scleral flap to prevent immediate hypotony. These subjective procedures provide a myriad of pressure excursions within the first week post-operatively. The MicroShunt is a fixed flow resistor and the pressure excursions are reduced to a standard deviation of ±4–5 mmHg which can be half that of the aforementioned filtering devices.

Potential early post-operative complications include hyphaema (Fig. 7.8), obstruction of the tube (Fig. 7.9), wound leak and hypotony. Transient numerical hypotony is the most common complication and can be managed with observation. If there is shallowing of the anterior chamber or large choroidal effusions,

Fig. 7.8 Hyphaema associated with the PRESERFLO® MicroShunt. (Copyright Chelvin Sng, FRCSEd; reproduced with permission)

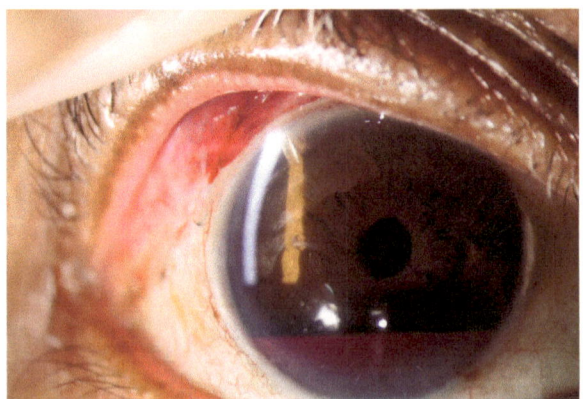

Fig. 7.9 Obstruction of
the PRESERFLO®
MicroShunt with (**a**) a
blood clot and (**b**) iris.
(Copyright Chelvin Sng,
FRCSEd; reproduced with
permission)

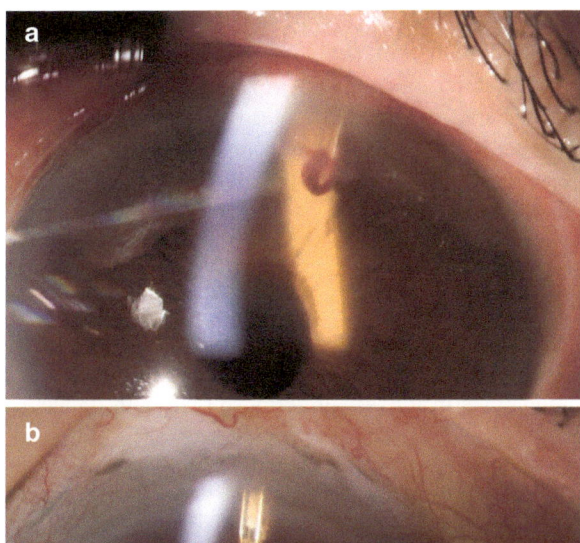

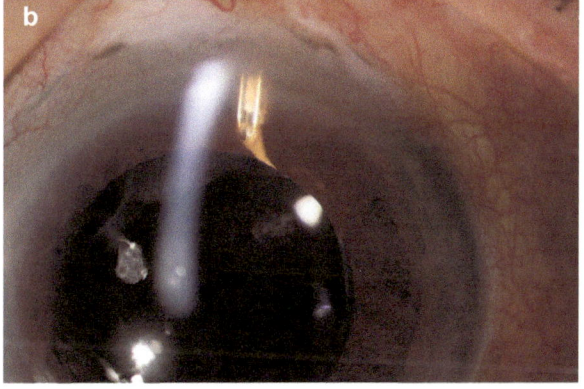

cycloplegics can be commenced and if necessary, injection of viscoelastic into the
anterior chamber can be performed. The patient should be observed closely for
intraocular pressure spikes if viscoelastic is injected into the anterior chamber. Tube
obstruction from iris is a concern if the internal end of the Microshunt is posteriorly
located and close to the iris (Fig. 7.9b), and YAG laser or a needle can be used to
remove iris from the tip if required. Obstruction of the tube with fibrin or inflammatory debris is usually transient and self-resolving with topical steroids. Wound leaks
may be present if conjunctival closure was inadequate. Leaks will usually settle
with conservative management, such as bandage contact lenses for anterior leaks.
Aqueous misdirection is rare with this device. Similarly, decompression retinopathy
has not been observed but is a theoretical concern if there is hypotony.

7.7.3   Late Complications

As with trabeculectomy, bleb encystment can occur and may require needling and/
or bleb revision. Both needling and bleb revision are typically performed with antimetabolites to modulate would healing. Erosion or migration of the shunt is

fortunately rare and can be managed with revision of the shunt and bleb. Blebitis and endophthalmitis have not been reported following MicroShunt implantation but are potential complications of any glaucoma filtration procedure which creates a bleb. Persistent hypotony on two consecutive visits beyond 90 days has not been reported. Lastly, corneal decompensation is a potential complication but this risk can be reduced by preventing the shunt or MMC from coming into contact with the endothelium.

7.8   Conclusion

The PRESERFLO MicroShunt is a promising new device that offers substantial reductions in IOP, rivalling those seen with trabeculectomy, in a less invasive and safer procedure. Its improved safety profile may permit earlier surgical intervention in glaucoma management.

References

1. Investigators A. 7. The relationship between control of intraocular pressure and visual field deterioration. The Advanced Glaucoma Intervention Study (AGIS). Am J Ophthalmol. 2000;130:429–40.
2. Anderson D, Drance S, Schulzer M. Comparison of glaucomatous progression between untreated patients with normal-tension glaucoma and patients with therapeutically reduced intraocular pressures. Am J Ophthalmol. 1998;126:487–97.
3. Chauhan BC, Drance SM. The relationship between intraocular pressure and visual field progression in glaucoma. Graefes Arch Clin Exp Ophthalmol. 1992;230:521–6.
4. Susanna R, De Moraes CG, Cioffi GA, Ritch R. Why do people (still) go blind from glaucoma? Transl Vis Sci Technol. 2015;4:1.
5. Cairns JE. Trabeculectomy. Preliminary report of a new method. Am J Ophthalmol. 1968;66:673–9.
6. Gedde SJ, Herndon LW, Brandt JD, Budenz DL, Feuer WJ, Schiffman JC. Postoperative complications in the Tube Versus Trabeculectomy (TVT) study during five years of follow-up. Am J Ophthalmol. 2012;153:804–14.e1.
7. Gerente VM, Regatieri CVS, Teixeira SH, Paranhos A Jr. Trabeculectomy learning curve: limbus versus fornix based conjunctival flaps—efficacy and complications. Invest Ophthalmol Vis Sci. 2007;48:844.
8. King AJ, Rotchford AP, Alwitry A, Moodie J. Frequency of bleb manipulations after trabeculectomy surgery. Br J Ophthalmol. 2007;91:873–7.
9. King A, Azuara-Blanco A, Tuulonen A. Glaucoma. BMJ. 2013;346:f3518.
10. Arrieta EA, Aly M, Parrish R, et al. Clinicopathologic correlations of poly-(styrene-b-isobutylene-b-styrene) glaucoma drainage devices of different internal diameters in rabbits. Ophthalmic Surg Lasers Imaging Retina. 2011;42:338–45.
11. Pinchuk L, Riss I, Batlle JF, et al. The development of a micro-shunt made from poly (styrene-block-isobutylene-block-styrene) to treat glaucoma. J Biomed Mater Res B Appl Biomater. 2017;105:211–21.
12. Lloyd MA, Baerveldt G, Nguyen QH, Minckler DS. Long-term histologic studies of the Baerveldt implant in a rabbit model. J Glaucoma. 1996;5:334–9.
13. Minckler DS, Shammas A, Wilcox M, Ogden T. Experimental studies of aqueous filtration using the Molteno implant. Trans Am Ophthalmol Soc. 1987;85:368.

14. Stokes K, Coury A, Urbanski P. Autooxidative degradation of implanted polyether polyurethane devices. J Biomater Appl. 1986;1:411–48.
15. Zhao Q, Topham N, Anderson J, Hiltner A, Lodoen G, Payet C. Foreign-body giant cells and polyurethane biostability: in vivo correlation of cell adhesion and surface cracking. J Biomed Mater Res A. 1991;25:177–83.
16. Pinchuk L, Riss I, Batlle JF, et al. The use of poly (styrene-block-isobutylene-block-styrene) as a microshunt to treat glaucoma. Regen Biomater. 2016;3:137–42.
17. Strickler F, Richard R, McFadden S, et al. In vivo and in vitro characterization of poly (styrene-b-isobutylene-b-styrene) copolymer stent coatings for biostability, vascular compatibility and mechanical integrity. J Biomed Mater Res A. 2010;92:773–82.
18. Pinchuk L. Biostable elastomeric polymers having quaternary carbons. Google Patents; 1998.
19. Pinchuk L, Wilson GJ, Barry JJ, Schoephoerster RT, Parel J-M, Kennedy JP. Medical applications of poly (styrene-block-isobutylene-block-styrene)("SIBS"). Biomaterials. 2008;29:448–60.
20. Acosta A, Fernandez V, Lamar P, et al. Ocular biocompatibility of quatromer (polystyrene-polystyrene triblock polymers) for glaucoma applications. Invest Ophthalmol Vis Sci. 2004;45:E-abstract 2929.
21. Acosta AC, Espana EM, Yamamoto H, et al. A newly designed glaucoma drainage implant made of poly (styrene-b-isobutylene-b-styrene): biocompatibility and function in normal rabbit eyes. Arch Ophthalmol. 2006;124:1742–9.
22. Beckers H, Kujovic-Aleksov S, Webers C, Riss I, Batlle J, Parel J-M. One-year results of a three-site study of the MicroShunt (R). Acta Ophthalmol. 2017;95:28–9.
23. Riss I, Batlle J, Pinchuk L, Kato YP, Weber BA, Parel JM. One-year results on the safety and efficacy of the InnFocus MicroShunt depending on placement and concentration of mitomycin C. J Fr Ophtalmol. 2015;38:855–60.
24. Batlle JF, Fantes F, Riss I, et al. Three-year follow-up of a novel aqueous humor microshunt. J Glaucoma. 2016;25:e58–65.
25. Santen Pharmaceutical. Santen Announces Topline Data for DE-128 (MicroShunt) Demonstrating Reductions in IOP and Medication Use in Patients with Glaucoma. Press Release, 30 Aug 2019. https://eyewire.news/articles/santen-announces-topline-data-for-de-128-microshunt-demonstrating-reductions-in-iop-and-medication-use-in-patients-with-glaucoma/. Accessed 18 Sep 2019.

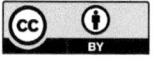

Suprachoroidal MIGS Devices

8

Julian Garcia-Feijoo, Jose Maria Martinez-de-la-Casa, and Lucia Perucho

8.1   Introduction

The suprachoroidal outflow pathway has the potential to reduce the intraocular pressure (IOP) dramatically, as the pressure gradient between the anterior chamber and the suprachoroidal space/uveal capillaries (colloidal osmotic pressure) permits flow even when IOP is very low. Compared with trabecular bypass minimally invasive glaucoma surgery (MIGS) devices, suprachoroidal MIGS harnesses a pathway that has a much greater IOP-lowering potential as suprachoroidal aqueous drainage is not dependent on the episcleral venous pressure. However, this pathway has a higher risk of severe and prolonged hypotony, because of the greater pressure gradient. The reason that most patients do not develop severe hypotony is because of fibrosis in the suprachoroidal space which restricts aqueous draining from the anterior chamber through the device from exiting the device into the suprachoroidal space. This may limit the long-term success of suprachoroidal devices [1].

8.2   Physiology of the Suprachoroidal Outflow Pathway

The natural suprachoroidal outflow pathway drains aqueous from the anterior chamber to the suprachoroidal space via the ciliary muscle [2]. Though the existence of this drainage pathway was proposed more than a century ago, it was poorly understood until monkey studies by Bill et al. in the 1960s allowed its physiology to be

J. Garcia-Feijoo · J. M. Martinez-de-la-Casa · L. Perucho (✉)
Department of Ophthalmology, Hospital Clínico San Carlos, Universidad Complutense de Madrid, Madrid, Spain

Instituto de Investigación Sanitaria del Hospital Clínico San Carlos (IdISSC), Madrid, Spain

Cooperative Research Network on Age-Related Ocular Pathology, Visual and Life Quality, Instituto de Salud Carlos III, Madrid, Spain

© The Author(s) 2021
C. C. A. Sng, K. Barton (eds.), *Minimally Invasive Glaucoma Surgery*,
https://doi.org/10.1007/978-981-15-5632-6_8

105

better defined [3, 4]. Aqueous permeates through ciliary muscle, the principal site of outflow resistance [3, 5], to the supraciliary and suprachoroidal spaces which exert a negative pressure. This outflow is IOP-independent over a wide range of IOP (4–35 mmHg) [3, 6, 7]. Aqueous exits the eye from the suprachoroidal space via two distinct drainage routes: the uveoscleral route (larger molecules: from the suprachoroidal space through the sclera to the orbit) and the uveovortex route (smaller molecules: from the suprachoroidal space to the uveal capillaries and the vortex veins). Of the two drainage routes, the uveovortex drainage pathway is the predominant pathway and is dependent on the difference in the colloid osmotic pressure between the uveal interstitial fluid (low) and the uveal capillaries (high) as well as the intraocular hydrostatic pressure [3, 8].

8.3   Early Surgical Approaches

It is surgically possible to bypass the ciliary muscle pathway, described above, by disrupting the attachment of the ciliary body to the scleral spur, hence allowing aqueous to flow directly between the anterior chamber and the suprachoroidal space. In 1905, Heine described a technique of cyclodialysis performed *ab externo* through the sclera using a spatula [9, 10]. Modifications of the technique were proposed in the twentieth century to prevent closure of the cleft, including the implantation of tissue or other material [11–13].

Unfortunately, these techniques caused significant ocular trauma and their efficacy in lowering the IOP was unpredictable with a high proportion of eyes developing prolonged hypotony followed by significant IOP spikes after spontaneous cleft closure, hence they were abandoned. Moreover, complications including suprachoroidal haemorrhage, hyphaema and secondary cataract were frequent. Nevertheless, this pathway is still unique in its impressive IOP-lowering potential, hence various modifications in the surgical technique of trabeculectomy [14, 15], non-penetrating glaucoma surgery [16] and glaucoma drainage devices [17] have been proposed over the years in vain attempts to utilize suprachoroidal drainage in addition to external filtration. Although these modifications did not result in higher complication rates compared with the conventional surgical techniques, neither did they improve efficacy.

8.4   *Ab-Externo* Suprachoroidal Devices

To avoid the complications associated with excessive filtration, some means of controlling the rate of aqueous outflow to the suprachoroidal space is required. Hence, several *ab-externo* suprachoroidal devices have been introduced, pioneered by the Gold Glaucoma Shunt (GGS, SOLX Ltd., Waltham, MA, USA) and followed by the STARflo Glaucoma Implant (iSTAR Medical, Isnes, Belgium) and the Aquashunt (OPKO Health Inc., Miami, FL, USA). Despite a sophisticated design incorporating flow control to prevent early hypotony with the GGS, long-term efficacy was poor as fibrosis and encapsulation developed around the device [18, 19]. Conjunctival peritomy and scleral flap dissection are also required in order to implant such *ab-externo* suprachoroidal devices, which added to the risk of scarring and, additionally, there was a concern that the GGS might also result in significant corneal endothelial cell loss because of its positioning. Hence, this has led to the development of *ab-interno* suprachoroidal MIGS devices, which are conjunctiva-sparing and less invasive.

8.5 *Ab-Interno* Suprachoroidal MIGS Devices

The emergence of MIGS has revolutionized glaucoma surgery [20]. The high safety profile of MIGS permits earlier use of surgery in the glaucoma treatment algorithm. Ab interno suprachoroidal MIGS devices are implanted through a corneal incision, hence spare the conjunctiva. Compared with *ab-externo* suprachoroidal devices, the potential advantages of accessing the suprachoroidal space with an *ab-interno* MIGS device are obvious, including less trauma, better safety profile and less inflammation and scarring. However, as with *ab-externo* suprachoroidal devices, the long-term efficacy of *ab-interno* devices may also be limited by scarring in the suprachoroidal space.

8.5.1 CyPass Micro-Stent

The CyPass Micro-Stent (Alcon Laboratories, Inc., Fort Worth, Texas, USA) was the first commercially available suprachoroidal MIGS device (Fig. 8.1). Originally developed by Transcend Medical, the CyPass Micro-Stent was a 6.35-mm polyamide tube with a 430-µm external diameter and a 300-µm lumen. After implantation into the suprachoidal space, it permitted unrestricted flow between the anterior chamber and the suprachoroidal space. The CyPass Micro-Stent had fenestrations (76-µm pores) along its length, to facilitate additional lateral flow and three retention rings at the proximal end, which acted as reference points for device position during implantation.

8.5.1.1 Surgical Technique
The CyPass Micro-Stent was inserted *ab interno* into the suprachoroidal space via a clear corneal incision. First, the device was loaded onto the retractable guidewire of the applier, assuming the same curvature as the applier guidewire, thereby facilitating insertion into the suprachoroidal space along the scleral contour. To obtain a good view of the anterior chamber angle, the patient's head was tilted away from the surgeon and the microscope tilted towards the surgeon. The device was inserted via a 20-gauge corneal incision diametrically opposite to the implantation site after pharmacological miosis and filling the target area with cohesive viscoelastic. The goniolens was placed on the cornea and the applier inserted through the corneal incision (Fig. 8.2). The blunt tip of the applier guidewire was slowly advanced

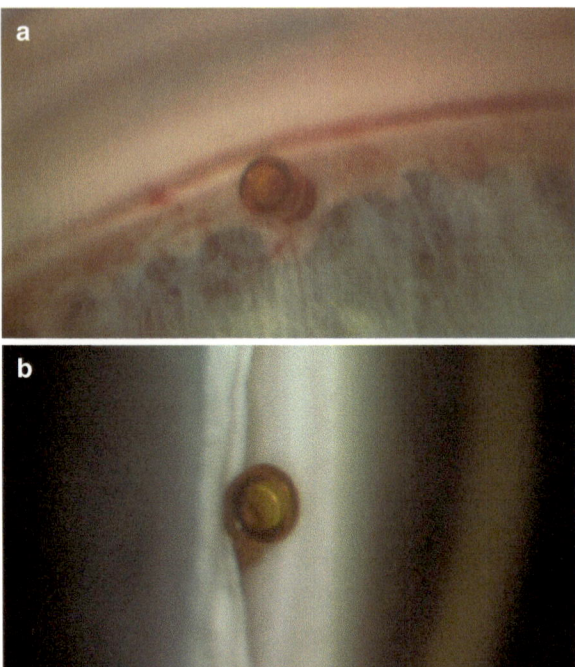

Fig. 8.1 (**a**) A CyPass Micro-Stent in a good position on gonioscopy in the operating theatre at the end of surgery. Note the blood outlining Schlemm's canal demonstrating that the collar of the CyPass Micro-Stent is sitting at the level of trabecular meshwork, well away from cornea and the entry of the CyPass Micro-Stent into the ciliary body band, peripheral to iris root (copyright Moorfields Eye Hospital and Keith Barton, reproduced with permission). (**b**) A well-positioned and patent CyPass Micro-Stent visible on gonioscopy a number of weeks after surgery (Copyright Moorfields Eye Hospital and Keith Barton; reproduced with permission)

between scleral spur and ciliary body, ensuring no iris movement when entering the angle. If the guidewire was inserted into the correct tissue plane and, if the insertion angle were correct, very little resistance would be encountered when inserting the device between ciliary body and sclera. The curvature of the applier guidewire permitted the CyPass Micro-Stent to advance along the scleral curvature. Once the CyPass Micro-Stent was at the correct depth, depression of the release button allowed the guidewire to retract. Ideally, the device was positioned so that the rim of the collar was at the upper border of the trabecular meshwork. After implantation of the CyPass Micro-stent, the viscoelastic was removed completely and the corneal incision sealed by hydration. A demonstration of the technique is available online (www.youtube.com/watch?v=_WXNL0CoJws&list=UUnkpnhwaQCC4Ary7gIyX RIw&index=2, accessed 2nd November 2019).

Poor Visualization of the Anterior Chamber Angle
Good visualization of the anterior chamber angle during implantation was important, though less critical than with trabecular meshwork stents as the target

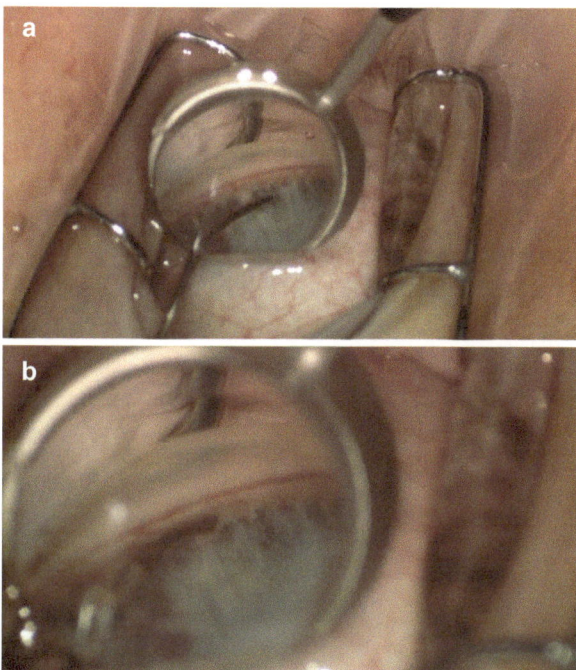

Fig. 8.2 (**a, b**) Insertion of the CyPass Micro-Stent in Fig. 8.1 (Copyright Moorfields Eye Hospital and Keith Barton; reproduced with permission)

implantation site, the ciliary body band is, on account of its position as the most posterior structure in the angle before the iris root, harder to miss. The CyPass was approved for implantation in eyes with open-angle glaucoma (Shaffer grade 3 or 4).

Resistance Encountered During Implantation

If resistance was encountered when advancing the device, this was either due to failure of the device to follow the scleral curvature or positioning of the tip of the guidewire in iris or ciliary body rather than between ciliary body and sclera. If the angulation and position of the applier were corrected, the device could be implanted in the suprachoroidal space with very little resistance.

Position of Device Too Anterior

If the proximal end of the CyPass Micro-Stent was positioned more anterior than the ideal position (rim of the collar at the level of the trabecular meshwork) (Fig. 8.3), the guidewide tube of the applier could be used to gently push the device deeper into the suprachoroidal space.

Position of Device Too Posterior

If the CyPass Micro-Stent was pushed too far into the suprachoroidal space, then there was a higher risk of post-operative device occlusion by iris. Sometimes the

Fig. 8.3 (**a**) Improperly positioned CyPass Micro-Stent protruding anteriorly and abutting cornea 2 years after surgery (copyright Moorfields Eye Hospital and Keith Barton, reproduced with permission). (**b**) The same CyPass Micro-Stent as (**a**), demonstrating that three rings are visible and the collar is very close to the cornea on gonioscopy, with a consequent high risk of corneal endothelial cell loss (Copyright Moorfields Eye Hospital and Keith Barton; reproduced with permission)

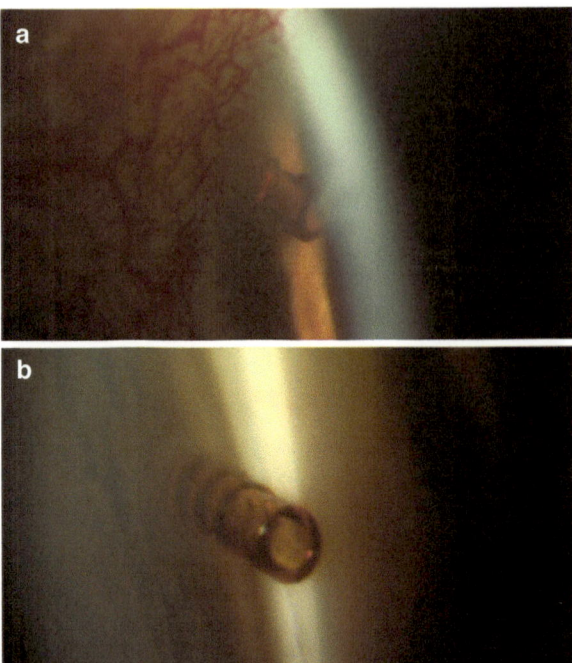

device could then be grasped carefully with retinal micro-forceps and pulled gently forwards into the anterior chamber. If the CyPass Micro-Stent were implanted so posteriorly that the tip of its collar could not be visualized, the device would have to be abandoned and left in the supra-choroidal space as attempted removal would cause excessive trauma. Implantation of a second CyPass Micro-Stent in the same eye would then generally be performed at least 2 clock-hours away from the first, in order to avoid the creation of a cyclodialysis cleft between the devices.

8.5.1.2 Mechanism of Action

Ultrasound biomicroscopy [21] and optical coherence tomography (OCT) [22] studies have shown that aqueous accumulated in the suprachoroidal space around and posterior to the CyPass Micro-Stent. In addition, as the device resumed a straight configuration after guidewire retraction, this created a fluid-filled space between the device and the sclera (tenting). Ultrasound biomicroscopy imaging of the suprachoroidal lake has shown that it could extend 360° circumferentially around the eye after CyPass Micro-Stent implantation. However, the fluid around and posterior to the device, as well as the space between the device and the sclera reduced with time, due to fibrosis in the suprachoroidal space. Given the ease with which choroidal effusions resorb with pressure elevation, it is most likely that aqueous from the suprachoroidal lake exits the eye via the choroidal and vortex venous system.

8.5.1.3 Efficacy

The safety and efficacy of the CyPass Micro-Stent have been investigated in several clinical studies, including one large randomized controlled trial.

Hoeh et al. [23] reported the 6-month outcomes of combined cataract surgery and CyPass Micro-Stent implantation in an exploratory multi-centre case series of 98 patients. The patients were divided into two groups based on whether their baseline IOP was uncontrolled (IOP $\geq$ 21 mmHg, Cohort 1) or controlled (IOP < 21 mmHg, Cohort 2). In uncontrolled patients (n = 57), the mean IOP was decreased by 37% ($p < 0.001$) and the mean number of glaucoma medications was reduced by more than 50% ($p < 0.001$) at 6 months. Patients whose IOP was controlled at baseline (n = 41) had a 71% reduction in the number of glaucoma medications.

A similar study by Höh et al. [24] reported the 2-year outcomes of combined cataract surgery and CyPass Micro-Stent implantation, with the patients again divided into those with uncontrolled baseline IOP (n = 23, IOP $\geq$ 21 mmHg, Cohort 1) and those with controlled baseline IOP (n = 59, IOP < 21 mmHg, Cohort 2). The IOP at 24 months was 15.8 ± 3.8 mmHg (37 ± 19% decrease from baseline IOP) and 16.1 ± 3.2 mmHg (0 ± 28% decrease from baseline IOP) in Cohort 1 and Cohort 2, respectively. The mean number of glaucoma medications at 24 months was 1.0 ± 1.1 in Cohort 1 and 1.1 ± 1.1 in Cohort 2. Fifteen subjects (11%) required additional incisional glaucoma surgery.

Garcia-Feijoo et al. [25] reported the results of the DUETTE study, a single-arm multi-centre study which examined the efficacy and safety of CyPass Micro-Stent implantation as a solo procedure in patients with medically uncontrolled POAG. Of the 65 patients recruited, 12-month data were available for 55 patients. At 12 months, there was a significant decrease in the mean IOP (16.4 ± 5.5 mmHg vs. 24.5 ± 2.8 mmHg, $p < 0.001$) and the mean number of glaucoma medications (1.4 ± 1.3 vs. 2.2 ± 1.1, $p = 0.002$). Nine patients required secondary incisional glaucoma surgery and two patients underwent implantation of a second Cypass Micro-Stent.

Vold et al. [26] reported the 2-year results of the COMPASS study (n = 505), a randomized comparative trial comparing stand-alone cataract surgery (control group, n = 131) with combined cataract surgery and CyPass Micro-Stent implantation (microstent group, n = 374). At baseline, both groups had similar mean IOP (24.5 ± 3.0 in the control group and 24.4 ± 2.8 mmHg in the microstent group, $p > 0.05$) and mean number of medications (1.3 ± 1.0 in the control group and 1.4 ± 0.9 in the microstent group, $p > 0.05$). At 2 years, a greater percentage of patients in the microstent group achieved $\geq$20% reduction in unmedicated IOP compared with the control group (77% vs. 60%, $p < 0.001$). The mean IOP reduction was 7.4 mmHg when combined surgery was performed and 5.4 mmHg when cataract surgery was performed as a standalone procedure ($p < 0.001$). At 2 years, 59% of the patients in the control group did not require any glaucoma medications compared to 85% of the patients in the microstent group. Three patients from the microstent group and four patients from the control group required further glaucoma surgery.

8.5.1.4 Complications

As a minimally invasive and blebless glaucoma surgical procedure, the CyPass Micro-Stent had a better safety profile than conventional glaucoma procedures such as trabeculectomy and tube shunts. The post-operative care was also less intense than that after the above procedures [27]. However, compared with trabecular bypass MIGS procedures, the CyPass Micro-Stent was associated with potentially more severe complications.

Intra-operative Complications

Serious intraoperative complications were rare with the CyPass. Typically a minor amount of bleeding might occur if the tip of the guidewire engaged the anterior chamber angle in an insufficiently peripheral position, catching the iris root. It was rare for bleeding to impede visualization for implantation but, when it did, injection of additional viscoelastic into the anterior chamber was usually sufficient to improve the view. There was also the possibility of inadvertent lens or corneal damage during implantation.

Significant lateral movement of the applier or an excessively traumatic implantation could have resulted in a cyclodialysis cleft around the CyPass, resulting in chronic postoperative hypotony.

Post-operative Complications

Inflammation

The incidence of early post-operative inflammation (within the first month) after CyPass Micro-Stent implantation has been reported to be around 4.2–8.6% and resolved in all cases without any sequelae [25, 26]. Hoeh et al. observed late-onset inflammation in 3.7% ($n = 5$) of his patients [28], whereas Kerr et al. reported 10% ($n = 2$), in theirs [29]. Notably, the two patients with late-onset inflammation reported by Kerr et al. had a history of uveitis.

Eyes with early or late-onset post-operative inflammation require an increased frequency of topical steroids, which can be titrated according to the severity of inflammation and may be necessary for several months. The IOP should be monitored closely in these eyes to identify and treat steroid responsiveness.

Hypotony

When post-operative hypotony occurred with the Cypass, it was the result of aqueous flow into the suprachoroidal space through the CyPass Micro-Stent or around the device (cyclodialysis cleft).

In the COMPASS study, hypotony occurred in 11 subjects (2.9%) undergoing combined CyPass Micro-Stent implantation with cataract surgery, with three cases considered clinically significant (i.e. associated with early maculopathy). Hypotony was transient in all 11 subjects and resolved spontaneously. Seven subjects in the microstent group developed a cyclodialysis cleft exceeding 2 mm, but none developed hypotony and did not require re-operation, so clearly were not functional clefts [26].

Hoeh et al. observed transient early hypotony in 13.8% of patients undergoing combined CyPass Micro-Stent implantation and cataract surgery. With the exception of one patient who took 6 months to resolve, the hypotony resolved spontaneously by 1 month [23]. Hoeh et al. also reported early hypotony in 14% of subjects undergoing combined CyPass Micro-Stent implantation and cataract surgery in another series, with all cases resolving spontaneously without visual sequelae or further surgical intervention [28]. A study reporting 2-year outcomes for CyPass Micro-Stent implantation in conjunction with cataract surgery found a similar incidence of early transient hypotony (15.4% of eyes), also resolving spontaneously in all cases [24].

When post-operative hypotony occurred after CyPass Micro-Stent implantation, the frequency of topical steroids would be reduced to encourage suprachoroidal fibrosis around the device. Rarely, hypotony persisted or was associated with hypotony maculopathy or choroidal detachment. In such cases, surgical intervention was occasionally required to occlude the Cypass Micro-Stent. Sii et al. [30] have reported two cases of persistent hypotony which were successfully treated by occluding the device's lumen *ab interno* with a 4-0 Nylon suture (www.youtube.com/watch?v=5zZnrSyB5vM&list=UUnkpnhwaQCC4Ary7gIyXRIw&index=11&t=0s, accessed 2nd November 2019).

The risk of hypotony was believed to be higher in highly myopic eyes.

IOP Spikes

IOP elevation in the immediate post-operative period (up to 48 h after the surgery) was most often due to retained viscoelastic and could be remedied by posterior lip pressure on the corneal incision using a hypodermic needle at the slit-lamp or medication. Less commonly, IOP elevation in the immediate post-operative period may have been due to occlusion with blood or iris. An IOP spike after the second or third postoperative week could be due to steroid responsiveness or occlusion of the implant or surrounding cleft with fibrosis (or both).

In the COMPASS study, 16 subjects in the microstent group (4.3%) developed transient IOP spikes, defined as IOP ≥ 10 mmHg above baseline values. All cases resolved, although three subjects required additional glaucoma surgical intervention for IOP control [26]. The frequency of transient IOP spikes was 10.5% in a study by Hoeh et al. [23] and 10.8% in a study by García-Feijoó et al. (defined as IOP > 30 mmHg that resolved either on its own or by adding glaucoma medications) [25]. Kerr et al. reported a higher rate of transient post-operative IOP spikes, occurring in 20% of subjects. Fortunately, none of these subjects required further glaucoma surgery or experienced a deterioration in best-corrected visual acuity (BCVA) [29].

Hyphaema

The frequency of post-operative hyphaema was reported at between 1.5% and 15%, with all cases resolving spontaneously within the first month [24–26, 28, 29].

Deterioration in Vision (Loss of ≥2 Lines of BCVA)

After CyPass Micro-Stent implantation, 1.1–3.1% of patients lost ≥2 lines of BCVA [25, 26, 28]. The causes of the vision loss included cystoid macular oedema, cataract progression (in phakic patients who underwent CyPass Micro-Stent implantation as a solo procedure), corneal oedema or posterior capsular opacification, with the management directed at each cause (e.g. cataract surgery, YAG laser capsulotomy).

Device Occlusion

Occlusion of the CyPass Micro-Stent with peripheral anterior synechiae (PAS) occurred in 2.1% of subjects in the COMPASS study [26]. García-Feijoó et al. reported that the device was occluded by PAS in two subjects (3.1%), and Nd:YAG laser was successfully used to clear the occlusion in one subject [25]. Hoeh et al. reported partial or complete device obstruction in nine subjects (5.4%), of which the device was occluded by PAS in two [28]. They also reported that occlusion occurred within the first 3 months in 80% of the 12 subjects (8.8%) in whom the CyPass Micro-Stent was occluded and was usually due to excessively posterior implantation of the device [24].

Device Malposition

Device malposition occurred in two patients and device migration/dislodgement occurred in two patients in the COMPASS study [26]. Hoeh et al. reported that one subject with an anteriorly positioned CyPass Micro-Stent required additional surgery to push the device further into the suprachoroidal space [23]. Kerr et al. reported that, in the hands of an experienced surgeon, device re-positioning can easily be performed at the slit lamp with a 30-gauge needle [29]. If the position of the CyPass Micro-Stent was too anterior after the surgery, it should be re-positioned as soon as possible before fibrosis and encapsulation develops.

Conversely, if the CyPass Micro-Stent was implanted too posteriorly in the suprachoroidal space, there was a higher risk of device occlusion by iris or PAS [28].

Additional Glaucoma Surgery

In the COMPASS study, three subjects (0.8%) in the microstent group required additional glaucoma surgery to control the IOP [26]. A higher glaucoma re-operation rate was reported by García-Feijoó et al., with 11 subjects (16.9%) requiring additional glaucoma surgery, mostly within the first 6 months. A second CyPass Micro-Stent was implanted in two subjects and the remaining nine subjects required subsequent trabeculectomy [25]. Hoeh et al. also reported that additional glaucoma surgery was required in 11.0% [15] subjects [28]. The COMPASS study included subjects with mild to moderate POAG on 1.4 ± 0.9 glaucoma medications at baseline, many of whom were medically controlled prior to medication washout [26]. On the other hand, in the study by Garcia-Feijoo et al., the mean number of glaucoma medicines at baseline was 2.2 ± 1.1, and all subjects were medically uncontrolled [25].

Corneal Endothelial Cell Loss and Corneal Decompensation

The COMPASS-XT study (a post-approval extension of the randomized clinical COMPASS trial) showed that patients who had undergone combined CyPass Micro-Stent implantation with phacoemulsification had a significantly greater reduction in endothelial cell counts than patients who had phacoemulsification alone, 5 years after surgery. Based on these findings, Alcon, the manufacturer, voluntarily withdrew the CyPass Micro-Stent from the global market in August 2018 (www.alcon.com/cypass-recall-information). The extent of endothelial cell loss in the COMPASS-XT study correlated with the number of retention rings visible on gonioscopy, hence the associated corneal damage was almost certainly a consequence of the device position in the angle. Endothelial cell loss was more prominent when two or more retention rings were visible in the anterior chamber. Though none of the patients developed clinically evident corneal decompensation, this was of concern because the US Food and Drug Administration (FDA) restricts the use of the CyPass Micro-Stent to adult patients with mild-to-moderate open-angle glaucoma in conjunction with cataract surgery. The safety of the device is particularly important in this group of patients who are conventionally treated with glaucoma medication. If the CyPass Micro-Stent should become available again in the future, it is likely that the manufacturer's directions on the surgical implantation technique would be amended to recommend a more posterior positioning, specifying that the device should not protrude, ideally above the trabecular meshwork or at worst, the Schwalbe's line. It would be less likely for significant endothelial cell loss to occur in these circumstances. Alcon may also consider extending the indication for the CyPass Micro-Stent to more refractory cases of glaucoma.

In an earlier study, Hoeh H et al. reported that the incidence of contact between the CyPass Micro-Stent and corneal endothelium was 1.2%, as a consequence of anterior device placement. None of these subjects experienced visual loss or required additional surgery, albeit with a short follow-up of 294 ± 121 days [28]. In another study by Höh H et al., device–corneal endothelial contact occurred in 3.7% of subjects [24].

If the CyPass Micro-Stent was positioned too anteriorly or if contact is detected between the device and the corneal endothelium, it was advisable to re-position the device in the early postoperative period. Within a few weeks, fibrosis develops around the device, preventing it from being easily re-positioned or removed. In such circumstances, the CyPass Micro-Stent could be trimmed using 23 gauge vitrectomy scissors, so that it does not protrude beyond the Schwalbe's line (www.youtube.com/watch?v=mRHdplofoBM&list=UUnkpnhwaQCC4Ary7gIyXRIw&index=5&t=0s, accessed 2nd November 2019).

Cataract Progression

In a multicentre, single-arm interventional study by Garcia-Feijoo et al., cataract progression occurred in 12.2% of phakic eyes 1 year after stand-alone CyPass Micro-Stent implantation [25]. Höh et al. reported that CyPass Micro-Stent implantation was associated with cataract progression in 2% of phakic eyes [24].

8.5.2 iStent Supra

The iStent Supra (Glaukos Corporation, San Clemente, CA, USA) is another *ab-interno* suprachoroidal MIGS device which has the Conformité Européene Mark (Fig. 8.4). It is a ridged curved tube made of heparin-coated polyethersulfone and titanium. The length of the iStent Supra is 4 mm, with an interior lumen diameter of 165 μm. The mechanism of action of the iStent Supra is very similar to that of the CyPass Micro-Stent.

8.5.2.1 Implantation Technique
The implantation technique of the iStent Supra is similar to that described above for the CyPass Micro-Stent. A 1.5-mm clear corneal incision is sufficient for the insertion of the iStent Supra.

8.5.2.2 Efficacy and Safety
Myers et al. [31] reported the efficacy of iStent Supra implantation combined with the implantation of two iStent Trabecular Micro-Bypass Stents and post-operative travoprost in patients with refractory open-angle glaucoma and previously failed glaucoma filtration surgeries. This case series reported the 4-year outcomes although it was originally designed to be a 5-year study. The mean unmedicated IOP at all visits was ≤13.7 mmHg (≥37% reduction from baseline). Among eyes without additional medication or surgery, ≥91% of eyes had ≥20% decrease in IOP on one medication compared with pre-operative medicated IOP at all post-operative visits. At 4 years, 97% and 98% of the eyes achieved IOP ≤15 and ≤18 mmHg respectively on one medication. Additional medication was required in six eyes, and none of the patients required additional glaucoma surgery. The most frequent adverse event was cataract progression (16% of the subjects) [31].

Fig. 8.4 iStent Supra (Copyright Glaukos Corporation, SanClemente, CA, USA; reproduced with permission)

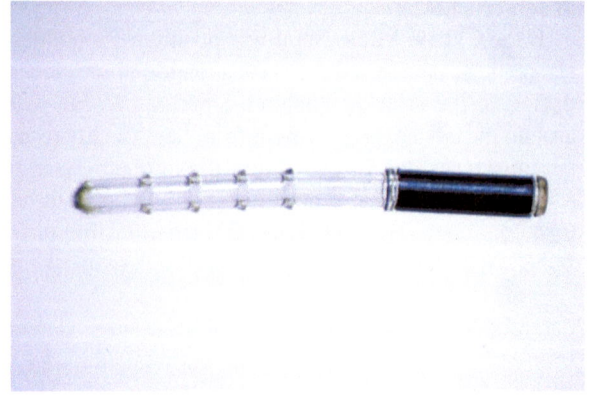

8.5.3   MINIject

The MINIject (iSTAR Medical, Isnes, Belgium) is the latest suprachoroidal MIGS device to be introduced (Fig. 8.5). Like its predecessor, the STARflo Glaucoma Implant (iSTAR Medical, Isnes, Belgium), the MINIject is made from STAR® material, which comprises of soft and flexible medical-grade silicone that conforms to the curvature of the eye. The STAR® material is composed of an organized network of hollow spheres with a micro-porous, multi-channel matrix which promotes bio-integration of surrounding tissues into the material, with the intention of reducing fibrosis and scarring, hence increasing the efficacy of the device. The MINIject is 5 mm in length and the green ring at the anterior segment of the device is used as a reference point for device position during implantation.

8.5.3.1 Implantation Technique
The implantation technique of the MINIject is similar to that described above for the CyPass Micro-Stent. The MINIject implant is preloaded in a transparent sheath attached to an applier handle, and sliding a wheel on the applier handle retracts the sheath back into the handle, leaving the device in place in the suprachoroidal space. Correct placement depth is achieved when the green ring is at the level of the scleral spur.

8.5.3.2 Efficacy and Safety
The first-in-human STAR-I trial for stand-alone MINIject implantation (Clinical-Trials.gov Identifier: NCT03193736) included 25 patients with mild-to-moderate POAG uncontrolled by topical glaucoma medications. Six-month data from the STAR-I trial showed a reduction in the mean ± standard error IOP (23.2 ± 0.6 vs. 14.2 ± 0.9, $p < 0.0001$) and the mean ± standard deviation number of glaucoma medications (2.0 ± 1.1 versus 0.3 ± 0.7), with 21 patients (87.5%) being medication-free and 23 patients (95.8%) achieving a minimum 20% IOP reduction from baseline. There were no serious adverse events related to the device or procedure and no additional glaucoma surgery was required. The mean central or peripheral corneal endothelial cell density was not significantly different from baseline [32]. At the time of writing, the 1-year data from the STAR-I trial have not been published.

Fig. 8.5 MINIject (Copyright iSTAR Medical, Isnes, Belgium; reproduced with permission)

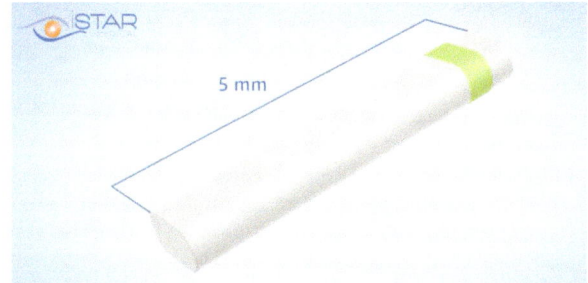

References

1. Bakharev AV, Fedorov AA, Batmanov LE. Comparative experimental morphological study of the impact of various drainages for cyclodialysis to adjacent tissues. Vestn oftalmol. 2008;12(2):44–6.
2. Johnson M, McLaren JW, Overby DR. Unconventional aqueous humor outflow: a review. Exp Eye Res. 2017;158:94–111.
3. Bill A, Phillips CI. Uveoscleral drainage of aqueous humor in human eyes. Exp Eye Res. 1971;12:275–81.
4. Bill A. The aqueous humor drainage mechanism in the cynomolgus monkey (Macaca irus) with evidence for unconventional routes. Investig Ophthalmol. 1965;4:911–9.
5. Alm A, Nilsson SFE. Uveoscleral outflow—a review. Exp Eye Res. 2009;88(4):760–8.
6. Bill A. Some thoughts on the pressure dependence of uveoscleral flow. J Glaucoma. 2003;12(1):88–9.
7. Yablonski ME. Some thoughts on the pressure dependence of uveoscleral flow. J Glaucoma. 2003;12(1):90–2.
8. Pederson JE, Gaasterland DE, et al. Uveoscleral aqueous outflow in the rhesus monkey: importance of uveal reabsorption. Investig Ophthalmol Vis Sci. 1977;16:1008–17.
9. Böke H. History of cyclodialysis. In memory of Leopold Heine 1870–1940. Klin Monbl Augenheikd. 1990;197(4):340–8.
10. Knapp A. The operative treatment of glaucoma by cyclodialysis. JAMA. 1909;53(10):765–7.
11. Barkan O, Boyle SF, Maisner S. On the surgery of glaucoma: mode of action of cyclodialysis. Cal West Med. 1936;44(1):12–6.
12. Barkan O. Cyclodialysis, multiple or single, with air injection; an operative technique for chronic glaucoma. Am J Ophthalmol. 1947;30(9):1063–73.
13. Jordan JF, Engels BF, Dinslage S, et al. A novel approach to suprachoroidal drainage for the surgical treatment of intractable glaucoma. J Glaucoma. 2006;15(3):200–5.
14. Lázaro García C, Benítez del Castillo JM, Castillo Gómez A, García Feijoó J, Macías Benítez JM, García Sánchez J. Lens fluorophotometry following trabeculectomy in primary open angle glaucoma. Ophthalmology. 2002;109:76–9.
15. Gupt S, Gupta V. Trabeculectomy augmented with ciclodialysis: a surgical option for refractory Glaucomas. J Glaucoma. 2016;25(7):e726.
16. Muñoz G. Nonstich suprachoroidal technique for T-Flux implantation in deep sclerectomy. J Glaucoma. 2009;18(3):262–4.
17. Ozdamar A, Aras C, Karacorlu M. Suprachoroidal seton implantation in refractory glaucoma: a novel surgical technique. J Glaucoma. 2003;12:354–9.
18. Hueber A, Roters S, Jordan JF, Konen W. Retrospective analysis of the success and safety of Gold Micro Shunt Implantation in glaucoma. BMC Ophthalmol. 2013;13:35.
19. Figus M, Lazzeri S, Fogagnolo P, et al. Supraciliary shunt in refractory glaucoma. Br J Ophthalmol. 2011;95:1537–41.
20. Saheb H, Ahmed II. Micro-invasive glaucoma surgery: current perspectives and future directions. Curr Opin Ophthalmol. 2012;23(2):96–104.
21. Gonzalez-Pastor E, et al. UBM findings after suprachoroidal CyPass implant for glaucoma: one year follow-up. ARVO; 2013.
22. Saheb H, Ianchulev T, Ahmed II. Optical coherence tomography of the suprachoroid after CyPass Micro-Stent implantation for the treatment of open-angle glaucoma. Br J Ophthalmol. 2014;98:19–23.
23. Hoeh H, Ahmed II, Grisanti S, Grisanti S, Grabner G, Nguyen QH, Rau M, Yoo S, Ianchulev T. Early postoperative safety and surgical outcomes after implantation of a suprachoroidal micro-stent for the treatment of open-angle glaucoma concomitant with cataract surgery. J Cataract Refract Surg. 2013;39(3):431–7.

24. Höeh H, Grisanti S, Grisanti S, Rau M, Ianchulev S. Two-year clinical experience with the CyPass micro-stent: safety and surgical outcomes of a novel supraciliary micro-stent. Klin Monatsbl Augenheilkd. 2014;231(4):377–81.
25. García-Feijoó J, Rau M, Grisanti S, et al. Supraciliary micro-stent implantation for open-angle glaucoma failing topical therapy: 1 year results of a multicenter study. Am J Ophthalmol. 2015;159:1075–81.
26. Vold S, Ahmed II, Craven ER, et al. Two-year COMPASS trial results: supraciliary microstenting with phacoemulsification in patients with open-angle glaucoma and cataracts. Ophthalmology. 2016;123(10):2103–12.
27. Gedde SJ, Herndon LW, Brandt JD, et al. Postoperative complications in the Tube Versus Trabeculectomy (TVT) study during five years of follow-up. Am J Ophthalmol. 2012;153:804–14.
28. Hoeh H, Vold SD, Ahmed IK, et al. Initial clinical experience with the CyPass micro-stent: safety and surgical outcomes of a novel supraciliary microstent. J Glaucoma. 2016;25:106–12.
29. Kerr NM, Wang J, Perucho L, Barton K. The safety and efficacy of supraciliary stenting following failed glaucoma surgery. Am J Ophthalmol. 2018;190:191–6.
30. Sii S, Triolo G, Barton K. Case series of hypotony maculopathy after CyPass insertion treated with intra-luminal suture occlusion. Clin Exp Ophthalmol. 2019;47(5):679–80.
31. Myers JS, Masood I, Hornbeak DM, et al. Prospective evaluation of two iStent® trabecular stents, one iStent SUPRA® suprachoroidal stent, and postoperative prostaglandin in refractory glaucoma: 4-year outcomes. Adv Ther. 2018;35(3):395–407.
32. Denis P, Hirneib C, Reddy KP, et al. A first-in-human study of the efficacy and safety of MINIject in patients with medically uncontrolled open-angle glaucoma (STAR-I). Ophthalmol Glaucoma. 2019;2(5):290–7.

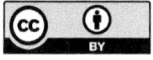

New Modalities of Cycloablation and High-Intensity-Focused Ultrasound

9

Natasha Nayak Kolomeyer and Marlene R. Moster

9.1   Introduction

Cycloablative or cyclodestructive procedures aim to lower intraocular pressure (IOP) by decreasing the function of the ciliary body and thereby decreasing the rate of aqueous production. Cycloablative procedures were typically used in refractory glaucoma in eyes with poor visual potential; however, more focused energy and targeted destruction of the ciliary body has led to an increase in cyclodestructive treatment options that are now an important adjunct to our surgical armamentarium.

9.2   Transscleral Diode Cyclophotocoagulation (TSCPC)

Cyclodestructive procedures have evolved since the 1920s, progressing from cyclectomy, cyclodiathermy, cyclocryotherapy, and eventually to cyclophotocoagulation [1–3]. Cyclophotocoagulation was initially performed in 1961 by using light from xenon arc photocoagulation [4] and subsequently using a ruby laser in 1969 [5]. Cyclophotocoagulation established a more widespread application once Nd:YAG (neodymium–yttrium–aluminum garnet) and eventually semiconductor diode lasers were developed. Nd:YAG cyclophotocoagulation (1064 nm wavelength) can be performed with or without ocular surface contact; however, noncontact methods were relinquished due to their higher complication rates. Currently, semiconductor diode lasers are the mainstay of transscleral diode cyclophotocoagulation (TSCPC). They have several advantages including greater uveal melanin absorption, compact size, and minimal maintenance requirements compared to prior lasers. Human cadaveric studies demonstrate epithelial coagulative necrosis and thermal coagulation of the ciliary stroma and vasculature in eyes receiving diode TSCPC [6].

N. N. Kolomeyer (✉) · M. R. Moster
Glaucoma Department, Wills Eye Hospital, Philadelphia, PA, USA

© The Author(s) 2021
C. C. A. Sng, K. Barton (eds.), *Minimally Invasive Glaucoma Surgery*,
https://doi.org/10.1007/978-981-15-5632-6_9

121

9.2.1 Procedure

• Typically, local anesthesia or sedation is administered along with regional (retro-bulbar/peribulbar/subtenon's) anesthesia.
• Common diode laser settings: Duration is often set at 2–3 s. Power starts at 1250–2500 mW. The power is titrated in 250 mW increments (maximum ~4000 mW) until an audible "pop" is heard; the power is then titrated to 250 mW below the "pop" threshold [3].
• The number of spot treatments varies between 14 and 20, sparing the 3 and 9 o'clock in order to avoid the long posterior ciliary nerves and vessels.
• The G-Probe is placed just posterior to the limbus, perpendicular to the limbus. This places the fiberoptic 1.2 mm posterior to the limbus. Maintain gentle pressure on the G-Probe throughout the treatment duration.
• Some physicians choose to administer a subconjunctival injection of steroids after TSCPC. The eye is patched and a shield is placed over the eye.
• Patients are placed on steroid drops after the laser, with the frequency of topical steroids titrated according to the severity of inflammation. All preoperative glaucoma medications are continued in the immediate postoperative period and can be selectively stopped depending on the IOP response. Patients are typically seen 1 day and 1 week postoperatively and subsequently depending on patient response.

9.2.2 Indications

TSCPC is indicated in patients with refractory glaucoma or a blind painful eye. It is typically used in patients with poor visual acuity (VA). It can also be used earlier in patients where incisional surgery is less ideal, such as those with significant medical conditions, bleeding diathesis, or scarred conjunctiva. The laser power for TSCPC may be reduced when treating eyes with good vision to reduce the risk of sight-threatening complications.

9.2.3 Results

A thorough compilation of the results and complications of TSCPC can be referred to in a recent review article; we have highlighted the most relevant findings below [7]. The treatment effect is often seen around 1 month after TSCPC; it is advisable to wait at least 1 month for retreatment if possible. TSCPC has demonstrated a range of effect on IOP (12.3–66% IOP reduction); post-laser IOP of ≤ 21 mmHg has been reported in 54–92.7% of eyes. Various studies suggest a correlation between IOP reduction and the amount of energy per treatment session or the number of laser burns. However, there are several studies that could not find a direct correlation. Other factors that influence treatment success include pre-laser IOP and the subtype of glaucoma. Lower success rates have been reported in aphakic, traumatic, and juvenile glaucoma. TSCPC success rates also increase with age and decrease with a history of prior surgery. More pigmented eyes usually require less energy, but there is no clear relationship with TSCPC success rates.

9.2.4 Complications

Adverse effects associated with treatment include vision loss (8.8–47%), hypotony (0–26%), hyphema (0–2%), anterior uveitis (9–28%), pupillary changes (0.8–50%), phthisis (0–10%), retinal detachment (1%), IOP spike, cataract progression, vitreous hemorrhage, lens subluxation, necrotizing scleritis, and rarely sympathetic ophthalmia [1].

The literature suggests a relationship between the amount of energy delivered and the risk of hypotony and phthisis [8]. It is unclear if this is a nonlinear relationship, but treatment sessions utilizing more than 80 J of energy tend to have higher rates of these complications. Glaucoma subtype (including neovascular glaucoma [NVG]) and high pretreatment IOP are also considered risk factors for hypotony and phthisis. This suggests that lower energy settings in a high-risk patient may be important in minimizing these complications.

Loss of more than two Snellen lines of VA was reported on average in 22.5% of eyes (0–55% range) [7]. Rotchford et al. evaluated the outcomes of TSCPC in patients with VA of at least 20/60. After 5 years, 73.5% of patients had an IOP of 16 mmHg or less and 30.6% had lost two or more Snellen lines of VA [9]. The proportion of patients who lost vision is consistent with that reported after incisional surgery, suggesting that TSCPC can be considered as an option in selected eyes with good visual potential.

Concerns regarding postoperative complications must be balanced against overall efficacy for each individual patient, as studies suggest a relationship between the amount of laser energy delivered and IOP reduction, as well as the risk of hypotony and phthisis.

9.3   Micropulse Transscleral Cyclophotocoagulation (MP-TSCPC)

The micropulse delivery mode of diode laser (MP-TSCPC, MicroPulse P3, IRIDEX IQ810 Laser System, Mountain View, CA, USA) is a more recent form of TSCPC. MP-TSCPC operates in an "on" and "off" cycle mode, delivering 810 nm infrared radiation from a diode source. During the "on" cycle, multiple bursts of laser are emitted by the device resulting in an increase in thermal energy absorption in pigmented tissues and induction of coagulative necrosis. Theoretically, the nonpigmented tissues do not cross the coagulative threshold because they have a lower rate of thermal energy absorption and are able to cool off during the "off" cycle. The MP-TSCPC also employs a novel probe that: (a) allows sweeping, continuous applications compared to individual spot treatments and (b) targets the pars plana rather than the pars plicata.

9.3.1   Procedure

- MP-TSCPC can be performed under topical, regional (peribulbar/subtenon's/retrobulbar), or general anesthesia. Some physicians find that topical or local anesthesia with a short burst of heavy sedation can be used without a need for retrobulbar anesthesia when in the operating room. However, if done in an office setting, regional (retrobulbar/peribulbar/subtenon's) anesthesia is commonly employed.
- Default laser settings are: micropulse mode, 2000 mW power, duty cycle of 31.33%, micropulse "on" time of 0.5 ms, and micropulse "off" time of 1.1 ms. At the surgeon's discretion, the laser is delivered over 360° for 100–360 s, while sparing the 3 and 9 o'clock positions as above for TSCPC. The duration of treatment is often titrated based on the patient's history. While the default laser settings are 2000 mW, more recently surgeons have titrated the power settings in the 2000–2500 mW range based on the patient's history as well.
- The MP-TSCPC probe is placed along the limbus perpendicular to the sclera. The probe is then moved in a continuous, sliding, slow motion around the limbus, sparing 3 and 9 o'clock, while applying firm pressure. The rate of movement is encouraged to be around 10–20 s per quadrant. The probe tip is designed to position the fiberoptic tip 3 mm posterior to the limbus (Fig. 9.1).
- Some physicians choose to administer a subconjunctival injection of steroids after MP-TSCPC.
- Topical steroid drops are typically applied four times daily post-surgery to control the inflammation and subsequently tapered as inflammatory response decreases.

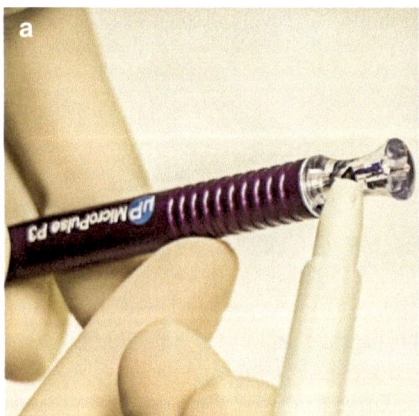
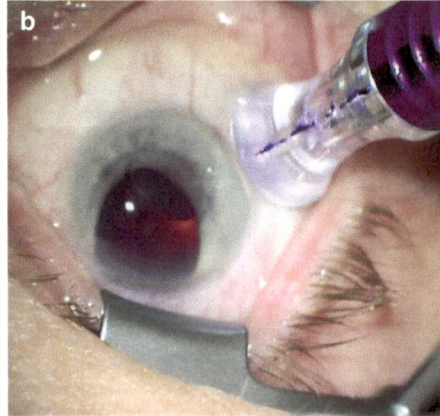

Fig. 9.1 Micropulse transscleral cyclophotocoagulation (MP-TSCPC). (**a**) The notch on the probe is to be placed toward the limbus. The notch is located on the rounder half of the probe and can be marked for easier visibility with a marker. (**b**) The probe is then placed with the marked notch perpendicular to the limbus. (Copyright Marlene Moster, MD; Bill Romano; and Natasha Nayak Kolomeyer, MD; reproduced with permission)

9.3.2 Indications

Indications for MP-TSCPC are broad, spanning noninvasive early interventions as well as refractory primary and secondary glaucomas. We recommend reviewing possible complications with the patient if using MP-TSCPC as an earlier intervention.

9.3.3 MP-TSCPC vs. TSCPC

MP-TSCPC versus TSCPC: A randomized exploratory study compared results of MP-TSCPC (with 100 s treatment duration) and continuous TSCPC in 48 patients with refractory end-stage glaucoma [10]. A successful primary outcome measure (IOP 6–21 mmHg and at least a 30% reduction with or without antiglaucoma medications after 18 months) was achieved after MP-TSCPC and continuous TSCPC in 52% and 30% ($p = 0.13$), respectively. There was a significant difference at 1 year (75% vs. 29%) that reached statistical significance ($p < 0.01$). Mean IOP was reduced by 45% in both groups from a baseline of 36.5 and 35 mmHg after 17.5 ± 1.6 months of follow-up. There was no significant difference in the number of IOP-lowering medications, while the complication rate was higher in the continuous TSCPC ($p = 0.01$) group including prolonged anterior chamber (A/C) inflammation, hypotony, and phthisis bulbi. There was a greater degree of IOP variance in the continuous TSCPC group, but the treatment settings were also more variable.

9.3.4 Results

Tan et al. [11] conducted a prospective case series of 40 eyes with refractory glaucoma that received a mean of 1.4 treatments of 100 s of MP-TSCPC. Eighty percent of eyes achieved relative success (IOP < 21 mmHg or reduction of 30% from baseline) with or without supplemental glaucoma medication, with 65% of eyes achieving successful IOP after one treatment. The average follow-up period of 17.3 ± 2.0 months was significantly longer than most other studies.

A retrospective review of 79 refractory glaucoma patients who received 120–360 s of MP-TSCPC demonstrated a treatment success rate of 75% at 3 months (IOP of 6–21 mmHg or a reduction of IOP by 20%), with an additional 10% of patients meeting the success criteria after the addition of IOP-lowering medications [12]. At 6 months, the treatment success rates dropped to 66% and were stable until the last follow-up for patients with at least 6 months of follow-up.

Emanuel et al. conducted a retrospective review of 84 eyes with a mean follow up of 4.3 months. There was a 41% and 53% reduction in IOP at 1 month and 3 months postoperatively, respectively [13].

Another retrospective review compared 320 s of MP-TSCPC results in nine pediatric (age 1–17 years) and 37 adult glaucoma patients [14]. At the 12-month follow-up period, success was achieved in 72% (26/36) of adult patients but only in 22%

(2/9) of pediatric patients ($p = 0.02$). Success was defined as IOP between 5 and 21 mmHg and ≥20% reduction from baseline at 12 months of follow-up without the use of oral carbonic anhydrase inhibitors, loss of light perception vision, or reoperation for glaucoma within the 12-month follow-up period. The mean IOP at postoperative months 1 and 6 was significantly decreased from baseline in the pediatric group, but the effect lost significance at 12 months. A majority (7/9) of pediatric eyes required reoperation to control IOP during the follow-up period.

9.3.5 Complications

The complications of MP-TSCPC in the retrospective review of 79 eyes by Williams et al. [12] included 7 patients with hypotony (9%), 21 (26%) patients with prolonged A/C inflammation, 13 (16%) patients with loss of two or more lines of best-corrected VA for ≥3 months, 4 (5%) patients with macular edema, 2 (2.5%) patients with corneal edema, and 2 (2.5%) patients with phthisis bulbi. There were no reported cases of mydriasis or loss of accommodation; however, given the retrospective nature of the study, this information was not directly elicited from the patients. The ten patients who underwent re-treatment did not seem to be more inclined to complications.

Tan et al. [11] did not observe any cases of hypotony or loss of vision after MP-TSCPC. All eyes had mild postoperative inflammation that resolved by 2 weeks in 90% of eyes and by 4 weeks in the remainder of eyes. Seven (17.5%) eyes with NVG developed hyphema. This study employed shorter treatment duration (100 s) compared to Williams et al. (120–360 s). Further studies would be required to ascertain whether there is a treatment duration related effect on outcomes and complications.

Emanuel et al. [13] observed 5 (6%) cases of persistent hypotony, 3 (4%) cases of IOP spikes, as well as hyphema (4%) and choroidals (1%). Persistent inflammation at postoperative month 3 was found in 74% of eyes. At postoperative month 1, 35% of eyes lost two more lines of vision. Three patients lost light-perception vision but were light perception at baseline. Tan et al. also found that MP-TSCPC caused significantly greater conjunctival inflammation and scarring compared to controls in Dutch Belted Rabbits, similar to continuous wave TSCPC [25]. Hence, further studies are required to investigate the effect of post-TSCPC conjunctival changes on future bleb morphology and survival.

9.4   High-Intensity Focused Ultrasound (HIFU)

High-Intensity Focused Ultrasound (HIFU) (Therapeutic Ultrasound System; Sonocare Inc., Ridgewood, NJ, USA) was evaluated as an alternative to ciliary body destruction in the 1980s [15]. Interest in HIFU initially faded due to the duration and complexity of treatment as well as significant complications (scleral staphyloma, phthisis, persistent hypotony, corneal thinning, and vision loss). However, modifications of the HIFU technology have resulted in recent renewed interest in this treatment modality. A miniaturized HIFU technique, ultrasonic circular cyclophotocoagulation (UC3, EyeOP1

HIFU, EyeTechCare, Rillieux-la-Pape, France), employs a circular operator-independent probe that focuses the ultrasound energy circumferentially on the ciliary body without operator movement. Unlike diode laser, focused ultrasound technology can treat a defined tissue volume at any depth or location within the eye, without being affected by pigmentation. The complex transducers and higher operating frequency allow for more selective treatment areas.

9.4.1   Procedure

- UC3 can be performed under topical, regional (peribulbar/subtenon's/retrobulbar), or general anesthesia.
- The coupling cone is placed in direct contact with the ocular surface and centered around the limbus. The coupling cone is then connected to a suction ring that establishes a low-level vacuum (70 mmHg) to maintain the cone in contact with the ocular surface to achieve alignment and control distance during the procedure. The probe is inserted into a coupling cone; probes are available in 11, 12, and 13 mm ring diameters (ring diameter size is determined preoperatively based on biometric data). The space between the ocular surface, the coupling cone, and the probe is filled with about 4 mL of room-temperature balanced salted solution. The probe (30 mm diameter, 15 mm height) is divided into six cylindrical piezoceramic transducers that generate ultrasound beams that allow treatment of up to 45% of the ciliary body. The ultrasound beam is focused at the depth of the ciliary body (2 mm below the sclera) [1] (Fig. 9.2).
- Each of the six transducers is activated for 4, 6, or 8 s (depending on treatment protocol), with a 20 s gap between each transducer, allowing cool down between each partial treatment. The entire treatment, which automatically proceeds with the activated foot pedal, is about 2.5 min.
- The settings specifically aim to avoid treatment of the retina, cornea, lens, as well as nasal and temporal zones.

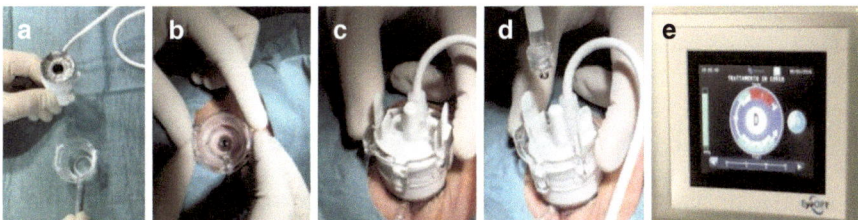

Fig. 9.2 Ultrasonic circular cyclophotocoagulation (UC3) procedure comprises two elements: the probe with the six piezoelectric transducers generating the ultrasound beam and the coupling cone (**a**). The correctly positioned cone must show a homogeneous ring of visible sclera; when this ring is regular, the cone is then maintained by a mild vacuum system (**b**). After verification of the effective suction, the probe is inserted and stabilized into the cone (**c**). During the procedure, the cone is continuously filled with saline solution (**d**), in order to allow the ultrasound transmission. The treatment starts in the superior sectors with a progressive activation of each transducer (**e**). (This figure and description have been reproduced from an open-access article by Mastropasqua et al. [1])

9.4.2 Mechanism

Ultrasound can cause thermal increase of up to 80 °C. The primary mechanism of action is reduction of aqueous production due to thermal necrosis of the ciliary epithelium. Histopathology studies in rabbits by Aptel et al. demonstrated focal necrotic changes in distal and intermediate ciliary processes, while sparing the basal and remaining parts of the ciliary body [15]. Untreated adjacent areas lacked signs of inflammation and had preserved architecture and vasculature. Additionally, there appears to be a correlation of treatment dosage and extent of ciliary process destruction [1]. Additional mechanisms of action could include modification of the scleral and conjunctival anatomy [16] and an increase in suprachoroidal and transscleral outflow [17–19].

9.4.3 Results

Giannacare et al. conducted a prospective multicenter interventional study of 30 eyes on maximum medical therapy with a 6-month follow-up [20]. Qualified and complete success (IOP reduction ≥20% and IOP ≥ 5 mmHg) was achieved in 70% and 46.7% of patients, respectively, while treatment failure was recorded in 6.6%. Eyes that were randomized to receive greater ultrasound exposure time (8 s per transducer) had greater IOP reduction compared to eyes with shorter ultrasound exposure time (4 or 6 s). There was significant IOP reduction on postoperative day 1 (39%) despite study protocol requiring discontinuation of ocular hypotensive medications in the immediate postoperative period unless IOP was above 21 mmHg.

The EyeMUST1 study was a prospective multicenter interventional study of 52 patients with refractory glaucoma [18]. Patients received either 4 s (group 1) or 6 s (group 2) exposure time per transducer (non-randomized). Success was defined as at least a 20% IOP reduction and IOP > 5 mmHg without additional hypotensive medications but with possible HIFU retreatment. Success was achieved at 6 months in 61.9% of group 1 patients and 65.4% of group 2 patients, while at 12 months the proportion was 57.1% and 48.0%, respectively (no significance at either time point). This difference was not statistically significant. Eight (15%) patients received HIFU retreatment. Twelve (22%) patients required a secondary glaucoma surgical intervention between 6 and 12 months post-HIFU.

Melamed et al. performed a prospective interventional study of 20 patients who received HIFU treatment (using 6 s exposure time per transducer), with 4 (20%) requiring retreatment [21]. Complete (IOP reduction ≥20% and IOP >5 mmHg) and qualified (allowance of additional medication and/or retreatment) surgical success was achieved in 45% and 65%, respectively.

Aptel et al. conducted a multicenter prospective clinical trial of 30 glaucoma patients without prior history of filtering surgery with a 6 s exposure time per transducer and 12-month follow up [22]. Complete success (IOP reduction ≥20%, IOP >5 mmHg and IOP < 21 mmHg with possible re-intervention and without additional hypotensive medication) was achieved in 47% of eyes and qualified success (allowance of retreatment without additional medications) was found in 63% of eyes.

De Gregorio et al. completed a prospective interventional study of 40 patients with an 8 s exposure time per transducer [23]. At 4 months, if the IOP was >21 mmHg with no adverse major complications related to HIFU procedure, the decision was made to retreat. Success was defined as IOP >5 mmHg and IOP < 21 mmHg without hypotensive medication and vision-threatening complications. Eighteen (45%) eyes achieved complete success with a mean IOP reduction of 44.3% at 4 months and 45.7% at 12 months. At 12 months, success was achieved in 85% of treated eyes with a maximum of three HIFU procedures.

9.4.4 Complications

Transient complications such as a fixed and dilated pupil (0–3%), anterior chamber inflammation (20–24%), superficial punctate keratitis (13–45%), subconjunctival hemorrhage (4–30%), corneal edema (7–20%), IOP spikes (0–7%), induced corneal astigmatism (0–3%), macular edema (0–3%), and hypotony (0–2%) have been identified [18, 20–23]. Loss of three or more lines of best-corrected VA was reported in 5–20% of patients [18, 22]. Notably, DeGregorio et al. noted scleral thinning in the treated sectors in 25% of eyes [23]. This evidence along with AS-OCT data suggesting scleral remodeling after UC_3 treatment highlights the importance of further analysis of the degree of scleral remodeling and how this may affect future filtration surgery. To our knowledge, there are no reports of persistent hypotony or phthisis after UC_3 treatment.

It is important to note that the UC_3 device requires suction to couple the device to the ocular surface, which increases the IOP for a period of 2.5 min. Although there are no reported cases of associated optic neuropathy, vein/artery occlusion, or visual field loss related to this specific device, this should be considered given the reports of LASIK-related complications [24].

9.5 Conclusion

Cycloablative treatment options for glaucoma continue to evolve. Recent developments such as MP-TSCPC and HIFU have improved safety profiles with variable results. We encourage the readers to balance the importance of safety and efficacy when choosing any surgical procedure, but especially a cycloablative procedure.

References

1. Mastropasqua R, Fasanella V, Mastropasqua A, Ciancaglini M, Agnifili L. High-intensity focused ultrasound circular cyclocoagulation in glaucoma: a step forward for cyclodestruction? J Ophthalmol. 2017;2017:7136275. Pubmed Central PMCID: 5420440
2. Pantcheva MB, Schuman JS. Chandler and Grant's glaucoma. 5th ed. Thorafore, NJ: SLACK Incorporated; 2013. p. 511–22.
3. Rand Allingham R, et al. Shields textbook of glaucoma. 6th ed. Philadelphia, PA: Lippincott Williams & Wilkins; 2011.

4. Weekers R, Lavergne G, Watillon M, Gilson M, Legros AM. Effects of photocoagulation of ciliary body upon ocular tension. Am J Ophthalmol. 1961;52:156–63.
5. Vucicevic ZM, Tsou KC, Nazarian IH, Scheie HG, Burns WP. A cytochemical approach to the laser coagulation of the ciliary body. Bibl Ophthalmol. 1969;79:467–78.
6. Schuman JS, Noecker RJ, Puliafito CA, Jacobson JJ, Shepps GJ, Wang N. Energy levels and probe placement in contact transscleral semiconductor diode laser cyclophotocoagulation in human cadaver eyes. Arch Ophthalmol. 1991;109(11):1534–8.
7. Ishida K. Update on results and complications of cyclophotocoagulation. Curr Opin Ophthalmol. 2013;24(2):102–10.
8. Vernon SA, Koppens JM, Menon GJ, Negi AK. Diode laser cycloablation in adult glaucoma: long-term results of a standard protocol and review of current literature. Clin Exp Ophthalmol. 2006;34(5):411–20.
9. Rotchford AP, Jayasawal R, Madhusudhan S, Ho S, King AJ, Vernon SA. Transscleral diode laser cycloablation in patients with good vision. Br J Ophthalmol. 2010;94(9):1180–3.
10. Aquino MC, Barton K, Tan AM, Sng C, Li X, Loon SC, et al. Micropulse versus continuous wave transscleral diode cyclophotocoagulation in refractory glaucoma: a randomized exploratory study. Clin Exp Ophthalmol. 2015;43(1):40–6.
11. Tan AM, Chockalingam M, Aquino MC, Lim ZI, See JL, Chew PT. Micropulse transscleral diode laser cyclophotocoagulation in the treatment of refractory glaucoma. Clin Exp Ophthalmol. 2010;38(3):266–72.
12. Williams AL, Moster MR, Rahmatnejad K, Resende AF, Horan T, Reynolds M, et al. Clinical efficacy and safety profile of micropulse transscleral cyclophotocoagulation in refractory glaucoma. J Glaucoma. 2018;27:445–9.
13. Emanuel ME, Grover DS, Fellman RL, Godfrey DG, Smith O, Butler MR, et al. Micropulse cyclophotocoagulation: initial results in refractory glaucoma. J Glaucoma. 2017;26(8):726–9.
14. Lee JH, Shi Y, Amoozgar B, Aderman C, De Alba CA, Lin S, et al. Outcome of micropulse laser transscleral cyclophotocoagulation on pediatric versus adult glaucoma patients. J Glaucoma. 2017;26(10):936–9.
15. Coleman DJ, Lizzi FL, Driller J, Rosado AL, Burgess SE, Torpey JH, et al. Therapeutic ultrasound in the treatment of glaucoma. II. Clinical applications. Ophthalmology. 1985 Mar;92(3):347–53.
16. Mastropasqua R, Agnifili L, Fasanella V, Toto L, Brescia L, Di Staso S, et al. Uveo-scleral outflow pathways after ultrasonic cyclocoagulation in refractory glaucoma: an anterior segment optical coherence tomography and in vivo confocal study. Br J Ophthalmol. 2016;100(12):1668–75.
17. Aptel F, Charrel T, Lafon C, Romano F, Chapelon JY, Blumen-Ohana E, et al. Miniaturized high-intensity focused ultrasound device in patients with glaucoma: a clinical pilot study. Invest Ophthalmol Vis Sci. 2011;52(12):8747–53.
18. Denis P, Aptel F, Rouland JF, Nordmann JP, Lachkar Y, Renard JP, et al. Cyclocoagulation of the ciliary bodies by high-intensity focused ultrasound: a 12-month multicenter study. Invest Ophthalmol Vis Sci. 2015;56(2):1089–96.
19. Aptel F, Dupuy C, Rouland JF. Treatment of refractory open-angle glaucoma using ultrasonic circular cyclocoagulation: a prospective case series. Curr Med Res Opin. 2014;30(8):1599–605.
20. Giannaccare G, Vagge A, Gizzi C, Bagnis A, Sebastiani S, Del Noce C, et al. High-intensity focused ultrasound treatment in patients with refractory glaucoma. Graefes Arch Clin Exp. 2017;255(3):599–605.
21. Melamed S, Goldenfeld M, Cotlear D, Skaat A, Moroz I. High-intensity focused ultrasound treatment in refractory glaucoma patients: results at 1 year of prospective clinical study. Eur J Ophthalmol. 2015;25(6):483–9.
22. Aptel F, Denis P, Rouland JF, Renard JP, Bron A. Multicenter clinical trial of high-intensity focused ultrasound treatment in glaucoma patients without previous filtering surgery. Acta Ophthalmol. 2016;94(5):e268–77.

23. De Gregorio A, Pedrotti E, Stevan G, Montali M, Morselli S. Safety and efficacy of multiple cyclocoagulation of ciliary bodies by high-intensity focused ultrasound in patients with glaucoma. Graefes Arch Clin Exp. 2017;255(12):2429–35.
24. Cameron BD, Saffra NA, Strominger MB. Laser in situ keratomileusis-induced optic neuropathy. Ophthalmology. 2001;108(4):660–5.
25. Tan NYQ, Ang M, Chan ASY, et al. Transscleral cyclophotocoauglation and its histological effects on the conjunctiva. Sci Rep. 2019;9(1):18703.

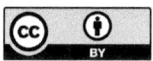

Controversies in the Use of MIGS

10

Georges M. Durr, Paola Marolo, Antonio Fea,
and Iqbal Ike K. Ahmed

10.1   Introduction

In this chapter, the discussion will focus on some of the "gray areas" that surround the use of minimally invasive glaucoma surgery (MIGS) in clinical practice. Many of the subjects covered review questions that physicians encounter when incorporating MIGS into their surgical practice. As a relative new-comer in the field of glaucoma surgery, these controversies highlight the challenges of implementing new technologies and future developments in an effervescent field of ophthalmology.

10.2   Phaco Alone Versus Phaco/MIGS, Is It Worth It?

Cataract surgery has a well-documented IOP-lowering effect [1–6]. Surgeons have often used this to their advantage in patients with glaucoma or ocular hypertension. With phacoemulsification (phaco) replacing extracapsular cataract surgery in the last two decades, the complication rates of cataract surgery have dramatically decreased, with excellent visual outcomes and rapid recovery. Currently, when a cataract is present in a glaucomatous eye, surgery may be offered in an attempt to

G. M. Durr (✉)
Department of Ophthalmology, Université de Montréal, Montréal, QC, Canada

Department of Ophthalmology, Centre Hospitalier Universitaire de Montréal (CHUM), Montréal, QC, Canada

P. Marolo · A. Fea
Struttura Complessa Oculistica, Città della Salute e della Scienza di Torino, Dipartimento di Scienze Chirurgiche, Università degli Studi di Torino, Torino, Italy

I. I. K. Ahmed
Department of Ophthalmology and Vision Sciences, University of Toronto, Toronto, ON, Canada

© The Author(s) 2021
C. C. A. Sng, K. Barton (eds.), *Minimally Invasive Glaucoma Surgery*,
https://doi.org/10.1007/978-981-15-5632-6_10

reduce IOP and improve the visual acuity simultaneously. With the advent of MIGS, the surgeon now has a variety of potential methods to assist IOP-lowering at the time of cataract surgery. The question is: is there really an added benefit of phaco/MIGS compared with phaco alone?

There have been numerous publications in the last few years, reporting the efficacy of MIGS in combination with cataract surgery, indicating an additional IOP lowering effect when compared with cataract surgery alone. In addition, there are a number of randomized clinical trials (RCT) addressing this issue [1–5]. On one hand, some large MIGS trials have shown that the additional IOP reduction conferred by MIGS is "only" 1.5–2.3 mmHg, with "only" 14–19.5% less eyes achieving an IOP reduction >20% compared with phaco alone [1, 3, 5]. Although the reported difference in IOP and success rate between phaco and phaco/MIGS seem small, these findings are still significant as they occur in the context of normal IOP, hence it is not as easy to show a difference between the two groups. Furthermore, proportional analyses of relevant clinical outcomes are important. For example, an increased proportion of patients in the MIGS groups compared to phaco alone remained medication-free at the end of the study period with differential rates varying between 13 and 35% [1–3, 5]. Some studies have shown that cataract surgery is more cost-effective when combined with MIGS than when performed alone [7], though more data are required to justify the additional MIGS procedure from an economic perspective. Another compelling argument is that phaco/MIGS results in fewer glaucoma surgical interventions later than with phaco alone. The HORIZON trial demonstrated that, at 3 years, a MIGS procedure could substantially reduce the requirement for later definitive glaucoma surgery in patients implanted with a Hydrus microstent (0.6%) compared with those who had cataract surgery alone (3.9%) [8].

It is difficult to account for surgical technique and verify accurate device placement in such trials. A well-targeted stent or a properly created trabeculotomy, which drains aqueous to a large aqueous vein (identified by looking at trypan blue outflow, increased trabecular pigmentation or blood reflux in the Schlemm's canal), is likely to enhance the IOP-lowering response [9]. A poor intra-operative view resulting in inappropriate device placement and a poor outcome can deter some surgeons. Better surgical training and more experience with different MIGS procedures are important in optimizing outcomes and maximizing the effect of MIGS implantation as an adjunct to cataract surgery.

The question remains as to whether this evidence of modest efficacy is truly clinically significant. From a patient's perspective, a reduction in drop load improves compliance, ocular surface irritation, and overall quality of life [10]. As poor compliance leads to glaucoma progression and increased costs to society, by implication adjunctive MIGS implantation should reduce both [11, 12]. At the time of cataract surgery, surgeons have a unique theoretical opportunity to improve a patients' quality of life and potentially delay progression or the requirement for future intervention. Above all, the high safety profile of MIGS gives surgeons more confidence in offering earlier surgery and this interventional mindset is now at the forefront of glaucoma therapy.

10.3   Trabecular Meshwork and Canal-Based Procedures: Cut Versus Stent Versus Dilate

MIGS options have broadened in recent years. Many of these target Schlemm's canal, a small 36 mm circumferential conduit with an inner diameter of 300–400 μm [13]. Currently, there are three main approaches to increase aqueous outflow via this conventional outflow pathway: cutting (ostomies) (Kahook Dual Blade [KDB, New World Medical, Rancho Cucamonga, CA, USA]); Trabectome [NeoMedix Corporation, San Juan Capistrano, CA, USA]; gonioscopy-assisted transluminal trabeculotomy [GATT]) with a suture, iTrack [Ellex Medical Pty Ltd., Adelaide, Australia] or OMNI [Sight Sciences Inc., Menlo Park, CA, USA]; and excimer laser trabeculostomy [ELT, Excimer Laser AIDA, Glautec AG, Nürnberg, Germany]), dilation (viscocanalostomy with iTrack or OMNI) and stenting (iStent Trabecular Micro-Bypass Stent and iStent *inject* [Glaukos Corporation, San Clemente, CA, USA] and Hydrus Microstent [Ivantis Inc., Irvine, CA, USA]) (Table 10.1). All of these procedures aim to reduce the primary resistance to outflow, the trabecular meshwork (TM), through cutting or stenting to bypass the meshwork or dilating Schlemm's canal to reduce resistance to aqueous transiting the canal to enter the collector channels. Success with these procedures depends on the presence of a functional distal outflow system (beyond Schlemm's canal) and on whether the healing response subsequently obstructs aqueous flow to Schlemm's canal.

Cutting techniques either incise, excise, or ablate the TM. The opening size of the trabeculotomy required to obtain optimal IOP-lowering is still under debate. Some earlier studies looking at outflow resistance have shown that there was only a small additional decrease (<10%) in outflow resistance with eyes receiving 360° of trabeculotomy versus 120° [14]. More studies are required to investigate the optimal trabeculotomy opening size required to achieve maximal efficacy in lowering IOP with the least amount of bleeding and postoperative hyphema. Upon review of current literature, hyphema occurs in approximately one-third of the eyes after GATT [15–17], ~9% of eyes after Trabectome [18–20] and ~8% of eyes after KDB [21–23]. Bleeding rates seem to decrease as the opening size of the trabeculotomy decreases. With regard

Table 10.1   Breakdown of the different procedures separated by the mechanism of action

Cut	Dilate	Stent
Kahook Dual Blade (New World Medical, Rancho Cucamonga, CA, USA)	iTrack™ (Ellex Medical Pty Ltd., Adelaide, Australia)	iStent Trabecular Micro-Bypass Stent and iStent *inject* (Glaukos Corporation, San Clemente, CA, USA)
Trabectome (NeoMedix Corporation, San Juan Capistrano, CA, USA)	OMNI®(Sight Sciences, Inc., Menlo Park, CA, USA)	Hydrus Microstent (Ivantis, Inc., Irvine, CA, USA)
Gonioscopy assisted transluminal trabeculotomy		
Excimer Laser Trabeculostomy (Excimer Laser AIDA, Glautec AG, Nürnberg, Germany)		

to cutting procedures, data on whether goniotomy (only an incision through the TM, e.g., GATT) or goniectomy (cut AND excision of the TM, e.g., Trabectome and KDB) procedures differ in a long-term efficacy and complication rates are lacking.

Dilation of Schlemm's canal alone may reduce resistance to aqueous outflow from Schlemm's canal to the collector channels as well as providing a gentle stretch to the TM [24]. Studies have shown that herniation of the collector channels with the elevation of IOP leads to decreased outflow of aqueous humor [25]. *Ab-interno* canal viscodilation is a relatively new procedure, and although previous studies of *ab-externo* canaloplasty have shown good results, the surgery is more invasive and requires conjunctival and scleral dissection to access the canal [26].

Stenting allows aqueous to bypass the TM, the main area of outflow resistance, and directly flow into the Schlemm's canal with less trauma to the meshwork or angle than the cutting procedures. The two available options for stenting are the iStent (iStent Trabecular Micro-Bypass Stent and iStent *inject*) and the Hydrus Microstent. Both these implants bypass the TM, with the Hydrus Microstent being a longer implant, which also scaffolds Schlemm's canal. The iStent is the smallest device implantable in the human body and can be placed at multiple locations in the canal. Large randomized control trials have shown that these implants are associated with a very low risk of complications. Current evidence indicates that the iStent *inject*, the first-generation iStent Trabecular Micro-Bypass Stent and the Hydrus Microstent, confer moderate efficacy in lowering IOP, either as solo procedures or combined with phacoemulsification [27–30]. The advantage of stenting procedures over the cutting and dilating procedures is that it creates a permanent communication for aqueous to flow from the anterior chamber to the Schlemm's canal. These stents can be obstructed by iris or peripheral anterior synechiae (PAS) (1–2%) [1–3], but elicit a much smaller inflammatory response than a cutting procedure and less blood reflux. Hence, theoretically, trabeculotomies are associated with a higher risk of PAS formation, hyphema, and membrane formation than stenting procedures.

Currently, there is no trial comparing the three approaches to Schlemm's canal. The choice of one trabecular bypass procedure over another depends on surgeon preference and expertise, cost, ease of access to the MIGS devices/procedures, and the relative risk of postoperative hyphema. Some may even consider combining stenting with dilation or dilation with ablation. The iTrack and OMNI devices allow a combination of canal dilation and TM ablation to be performed. Based on our clinical experience, it is likely that viscodilation of the canal decreases the incidence of postoperative hyphema by tamponading the reflux bleeding. Stenting, however, remains the least invasive trabecular bypass procedure with the lowest incidence of complications. Regardless of the surgery chosen, it is important that the surgeon is well-trained in the procedure, so as to achieve optimal efficacy with a low rate of complications.

10.4   Endothelial Cell Loss and MIGS

The COMPASS-XT trial (an extension of the COMPASS trial) uncovered a significant safety issue with the CyPass Micro-stent (Alcon Laboratories Inc., Fort Worth, Tx, USA) [4, 31]. This led to Alcon's voluntary withdrawal of the device from the market due to concerns of a significant increase in endothelial cell loss (ECL) compared to patients who underwent cataract surgery alone after a 5-year follow-up. The only factor that correlated with ECL was the position of the device in the angle. The more retention rings that were visible on the CyPass Micro-Stent, the higher the likelihood of significant ECL [32]. Importantly, depending on the angle anatomy, a device with one ring visible can still be at risk of causing ECL if it remains in close proximity to the endothelium. This emphasizes the importance of correct device positioning, especially for suprachoroidal devices.

MIGS addresses a void in the conventional glaucoma treatment algorithm, which exists between topical drops/laser procedures and conventional glaucoma filtration surgery (trabeculectomy and tube implants). The high safety profile of MIGS is an important characteristic that allows it to be offered earlier in the glaucoma treatment algorithm, either in combination with cataract surgery or as a standalone procedure. The recent finding of increased ECL with the CyPass Micro-Stent led to a review of all the current MIGS procedures and their risk to the corneal endothelium. Fortunately, to date, no other MIGS device (iStent Trabecular Micro-Bypass Stent, iStent *inject*, Hydrus Microstent, Trabectome) is associated with an increase in ECL compared to cataract surgery alone (Table 10.2). In contrast, previous studies have reported ECL between 8.0 and 18.6% at 2 years for tube shunts and between 9.5 and 28.0% at 1 year and 9.9% at 2 years for trabeculectomy [33–41].

Much is still unknown with regard to MIGS and its effect on the corneal endothelium as well as the effect of cataract surgery and conventional glaucoma surgery on the cornea. Several factors, including device material, aqueous humor dynamics, and inflammatory mediators have been hypothesized to play a role in ECL after surgery. It is clear from the COMPASS-XT results that the further away the device is positioned from the endothelium, the lower the risk of ECL. Hence, the likely cause for ECL is mechanical trauma to the corneal endothelium by the device. Trabecular bypass MIGS devices (Hydrus Microstent and iStent) are located away from the corneal endothelium when correctly implanted in the angle, and early data show that they are not associated with an increase in ECL [42, 43]. Dilating or cutting procedures (GATT, OMNI, iTrack, KDB) are unlikely to increase ECL (apart from the initial trauma from the surgery) as they do not require a device to be permanently implanted in the eye, although this remains to be confirmed [44].

Subconjunctival MIGS devices such as the XEN Gel Implant (Allergan plc, Dublin, Ireland) and PRESERFLO MicroShunt (Santen Pharmaceutical Co. Ltd., Osaka, Japan) are bleb-forming procedures which are more effective in lowering IOP, hence are typically reserved for patients who need a greater reduction in intraocular pressure. The risk-benefit profile of patients who undergo subconjunctival MIGS device implantation differs from that of patients who undergo trabecular bypass or suprachoroidal MIGS device implantation. Similar to trabeculectomy and tube implants, subconjunctival MIGS devices are often used in the context of more advanced glaucoma, and hence, there is a higher tolerance and acceptance of potential complications in exchange for higher efficacy in lowering the IOP and preventing glaucoma progression. Only one study has examined ECL after implantation of the XEN Gel Implant and showed no significant change in endothelial cell count

Table 10.2 Comparison of ECL rates between different MIGS procedures (adapted from reference [3])

MIGS procedures	N	Follow-up time	Mean % ECL	% with ECL > 30%
Schlemm Canal				
iStent inject (Glaukos Corporation)	505	24 months	13.1% treatment 12.3% control	10.4% treatment 9.5% control
	20[a]	12 months	13.2%	
Hydrus Microstent (Ivantis, Inc.)	556	24 months	14.0% treatment 10.0% control	13.6% treatment 7.2% control
		36 months	15.0% treatment 11.0% control	14.0% treatment 10.2% control
Trabectome (NeoMedix Corporation)	80[b]	12 months	No change	
Kahook Dual Blade (New World Medical)	Unknown			
Ab-interno Canaloplasty (Ellex Medical Pty Ltd)	Unknown			
OMNI (Sight Sciences, Inc.)	Unknown			
Supraciliary				
CyPass Micro-Stent (Alcon Laboratories, Inc.)	253	60 months	1 8.4% treatment 7.5% control	27.2% treatment 10.0% control
iStent Supra (Glaukos Corporation)	Unknown			
Subconjunctival				
XEN Gel Implant (Allergan plc)	11[c]	12 months	No change (+3.6%)	
PRESERFLO MicroShunt (Santen Pharmaceutical Co. Ltd.)	Unknown			

N = number of patients, ECL = endothelial cell loss, MIGS = microinvasive glaucoma surgery
[a]Arriola-Villalobos et al. [43]
[b]Maeda et al. [44]
[c]Fea et al. [45]

after 1 year [45]. We hypothesize that the risk of progressive endothelial trauma is minimized by a properly positioned implant, which is parallel to the iris and enters the eye posteriorly to Schwalbe's line.

10.5 Is the Suprachoroidal Space Dead?

The supraciliary space has long been targeted with the aim of decreasing IOP and attempts to access suprachoroidal drainage date back to the 1930s with the use of horsehair to increase suprachoroidal aqueous outflow [46]. Several features of this space make it an alluring target for surgical therapy. Firstly, the uveoscleral pathway accounts for 20–54% of the aqueous humor outflow in a normal eye and this decreases with age, with the main restriction to aqueous flow arising from the ciliary muscle [47, 48]. Secondly, there is a proven increase in uveoscleral outflow when drugs such as cholinergics and prostaglandin analogs are administered. Prostaglandin analogs are now the mainstay of topical glaucoma therapy due to their significant efficacy in reducing IOP [47, 48]. Finally, traumatic cyclodialysis clefts may profoundly reduce IOP without bleb formation and this reduction can last for many years [47, 48]. Unlike Schlemm's canal which is lined with endothelial cells, the suprachoroidal space is lined with myofibroblasts which predispose to fibrosis and scarring, hence the efficacy of suprachoroidal aqueous outflow in lowering IOP is more unpredictable. The advantages of draining aqueous to the suprachoroidal space include its size (indicating a large capacity for aqueous drainage) and, unlike the conventional aqueous outflow pathway, the reduction in IOP is not limited by the episcleral venous pressure.

These factors have resulted in the introduction of various implants and procedures to create and maintain a cyclodialysis cleft [49–53]. The disadvantages of previous suprachoroidal procedures or devices include high rates of intraoperative and postoperative bleeding, unpredictable efficacy in reducing IOP, hypotony, and sudden IOP spikes when the cleft closes. Biocompatible materials have been used to create a scaffold within the suprachoroidal space, creating a direct communication between the anterior chamber and the suprachoroidal space. The Gold Glaucoma Shunt (GGS, SOLX Ltd., Waltham, MA, USA) [54] and the STARflo Glaucoma Implant (iStar Medical, Isnes, Belgium) [55] are *ab-externo* suprachoroidal devices which require conjunctival as well as scleral dissection for implantation. Clinical data on the STARflo are limited, while the GGS has been associated with poor surgical outcomes [54]. Hence, the *ab-externo* approach to the suprachoroidal space has been abandoned for newer techniques utilizing an *ab-interno* approach. Until recently, there was only one commercially available *ab-interno* suprachoroidal MIGS device, the CyPass Micro-Stent (Alcon Laboratories Inc., Fort Worth, Tx, USA). The withdrawal of the CyPass Micro-Stent due to concerns of long-term ECL evident in the 5-year results of the COMPASS-XT trial has cast doubts on whether this space is a viable option after all [56, 57]. However, the ECL associated with the CyPass Micro-Stent is likely due to the position of the device in the angle causing mechanical trauma to the corneal endothelium and does not appear to be a consequence of suprachoroidal aqueous drainage. Thus, it is important for suprachoroidal and other intraocular devices to be positioned away from the cornea, preferably parallel to the iris.

Compared to MIGS devices targeting the Schlemm's canal, suprachoroidal aqueous drainage can potentially reduce IOP to a dramatic extent as the resultant IOP is not limited by the episcleral venous pressure. Surgical implantation of suprachoroidal devices is also technically easier compared with the implantation of trabecular bypass devices. The disadvantages of suprachoroidal aqueous drainage include unpredictable efficacy in reducing IOP and postoperative fibrosis or scarring which can result in a sudden IOP spike. For refractory eyes which lack healthy and mobile conjunctiva, suprachoroidal aqueous drainage provides a viable alternative to further conjunctival filtration surgery [58]. In addition, suprachoroidal MIGS devices can be combined with devices or procedures which utilize other routes of aqueous drainage (conventional aqueous outflow pathway and subconjunctival drainage) to achieve better IOP control.

The iStent Suprachoroidal Bypass System (iStent Supra, Glaukos Corporation, San Clemente, CA, USA) is another microstent that is in development with limited data available [59]. A further device currently under investigation, the MINIject™ (iStar Medical, Isnes, Belgium), is composed of a biocompatible silicone implant with micropores, the same material as the STARflo device. The advantage of this material lies in its ability to biointegrate in the suprachoroidal space. Currently, a randomized clinical trial (NCT03193736) is underway to evaluate the efficacy and safety of the MINIject, with clinical data reported at 6, 12, and 24 months. Preliminary results show a 39% reduction in IOP with mean IOP of 14.2 mmHg at 6 months, with 87.5% of patients being medication-free [60]. Although the suprachoroidal space is not well understood and much remains to be discovered about the optimization and maintenance of suprachoroidal aqueous drainage, current and new technologies on the horizon are promising.

10.6 The Great Debate: Subconjunctival MIGS and Trabeculectomy

Trabeculectomy is a time-tested glaucoma filtration surgery with multiple studies reporting long-term data substantiating its efficacy in reducing IOP by creating a filtering bleb [61–65]. However, this surgery is associated with a significant risk of complications and unpredictable results. Postoperative bleb management is complex, requiring many interventions (e.g., bleb needling and scleral flap suture removal) and visual rehabilitation can be prolonged. The success of trabeculectomy is highly dependent on surgical expertise as well as patient characteristics, with the creation of the scleral flap, suture tension, timing of suture–lysis, and conjunctival closure all having a significant impact on surgical outcomes. Furthermore, trabeculectomy is associated with a significant risk of complications, including hypotony, bleb leaks, and suprachoroidal hemorrhage. *Ab-interno* and *ab-externo* subconjunctival MIGS devices can potentially reduce the rate of complications, improve the predictability of surgical outcomes, and accelerate postoperative recovery. The efficacy of these procedures in reducing IOP has been a topic of debate in the glaucoma community and more prospective multicenter randomized trials are needed to compare the outcome of these devices with trabeculectomy.

The XEN Gel Implant is a 6-mm implant made of porcine gelatin cross-linked with glutaraldehyde, with an internal lumen diameter of 45 μm. It is implanted *ab interno* through a clear corneal incision into the subconjunctival space to create a filtering bleb, bypassing the TM [66, 67]. The length and the inner lumen of the device confer 6–8 mmHg of outflow resistance according to the Hagen-Poiseuille equation, hence protecting against hypotony. Despite the theoretical advantages of this approach, surgical outcomes can still be unpredictable. This is because microstents, which have a small lumen size, are at an increased risk of distal obstruction by tenon's capsule or fibrosis, or internal obstruction by pigment, heme, or fibrin. A large retrospective comparison of the XEN Gel Implant and trabeculectomy showed no difference in the failure rates and a similar safety profile between the two procedures [67]. In an attempt to position the implant consistently under the Tenon's capsule and to ensure that it is not occluded by the Tenon's, some surgeons prefer *ab-externo* implantation of the device with conjunctival peritomy or a trans-conjunctival approach to surgical implantation. Currently, no data are available comparing the different surgical approaches.

The PRESERFLO MicroShunt is a new subconjunctival MIGS device which is 8.5 mm long, with an internal lumen diameter of 70 μm. It is made of an inert bio-compatible biomaterial called poly(styrene-block-isobutylene-block-styrene), or "SIBS" [68]. The MicroShunt requires conjunctival and Tenon's layer dissection to properly position the implant in the anterior chamber and under Tenon's. Early data from Batlle et al. show promising results in a small sample of patients [69].

Ab-externo XEN implantation and the surgical technique of the PRESERFLO MicroShunt both involve conjunctival peritomy to ensure optimal device placement under Tenon's capsule, but there are a few inherent differences between the two implants. The MicroShunt was designed to be implanted *ab externo*; hence, some features of the device are more adapted to that placement. Firstly, the fixation fins prevent migration of the device and limit peritubular flow. The XEN Gel Implant is injected through a needle, which creates a larger track allowing peritubular flow, resulting in a higher incidence of early postoperative hypotony. The MicroShunt lumen is larger than the XEN Gel Implant and it is a longer and stiffer device. As a longer segment of the MicroShunt is located in the anterior chamber compared with the XEN Gel Implant, it may be more likely to damage the corneal endothelium or be in contact with the iris. Both implants are made of non-inflammatory and bio-compatible material (SIBS for the PRESERFLO MicroShunt and crosslinked porcine gelatin for the XEN Gel Implant).

Subconjunctival MIGS devices control aqueous outflow into the subconjunctival space to form a filtering bleb with potentially fewer complications and a more uneventful postoperative course. The efficacy of these novel devices is potentially comparable to trabeculectomy, with a lower risk of complications and more predictable outcomes. Whether these subconjunctival MIGS devices will eventually replace trabeculectomy or be used earlier in the glaucoma treatment paradigm remains to be seen.

References

1. Samuelson TW, Katz LJ, Wells JM, et al. Randomized evaluation of the trabecular micro-bypass stent with phacoemulsification in patients with glaucoma and cataract. Ophthalmology. 2011;118:459–67.
2. Pfeiffer N, Garcia Feijoo JG, Martinez JM, et al. A randomized trial of a Schlemm's canal mic-rostent with phacoemulsification for reduction of intraocular pressure in open angle glaucoma. Ophthalmology. 2015;122:1283–93.
3. Samuelson TW, Chang DF, Marquis R, Flowers B, Lim KS, Ahmed IIK, Jampel HD, Aung T, Crandall AS, Singh K, HORIZON Investigators. A Schlemm Canal Microstent for intraocular pressure reduction in primary open-angle glaucoma and cataract: the HORIZON Study. Ophthalmology. 2019;126:29–37.

4. Vold S, Ahmed II, Craven ER, et al. Two-year COMPASS trial results: supraciliary microstenting with phacoemulsification in patients with open-angle glaucoma and cataracts. Ophthalmology. 2016;123:2103–12.
5. Samuelson TW, Sarkisian SR Jr, Lubeck DM, Stiles MC, Duh YJ, Romo EA, Giamporcaro JE, Hornbeak DM, Katz LJ, iStent inject Study Group. Prospective, randomized, controlled pivotal trial of an ab interno implanted trabecular micro-bypass in primary open-angle glaucoma and cataract: two-year results. Ophthalmology. 2019;126(6):811–21.
6. Mansberger SL, Gordon MO, Jampel H, Bhorade A, Brandt JD, Wilson B, Kass MA, Ocular Hypertension Treatment Study Group. Reduction in intraocular pressure after cataract extraction: the Ocular Hypertension Treatment Study. Ophthalmology. 2012;119(9):1826–31.
7. Patel V, Ahmed I, Podbielski D, Falvey H, Murray J, Goeree R. Cost-effectiveness analysis of standalone trabecular micro-bypass stents in patients with mild-to-moderate open-angle glaucoma in Canada. J Med Econ. 2019;22(4):390–401.
8. Ivantis Announces Groundbreaking 3 Year Results from FDA Clinical Trial; First Device in Minimally Invasive Glaucoma Surgical (MIGS) Category to Demonstrate Significant Long Term Reduction of Severe Major Surgeries for Glaucoma Patients. https://www.prnewswire.com/news-releases/ivantis-announces-groundbreaking-3-year-results-from-fda-clinical-trial-first-device-in-minimally-invasive-glaucoma-surgical-migs-category-to-demonstrate-significant-long-term-reduction-of-severe-major-surgeries-for-glaucoma-pa-300842527.html?tc=eml_cleartime
9. Huang AS, Saraswathy S, Dastiridou A, Begian A, Mohindroo C, Tan JC, Francis BA, Hinton DR, Weinreb RN. Aqueous angiography-mediated guidance of trabecular bypass improves angiographic outflow in human enucleated eyes. Invest Ophthalmol Vis Sci. 2016;57(11):4558–65.
10. Gazzard G, Konstantakopoulou E, Garway-Heath D, Garg A, Vickerstaff V, Hunter R, Ambler G, Bunce C, Wormald R, Nathwani N, Barton K, Rubin G, Buszewicz M, LiGHT Trial Study Group. Selective laser trabeculoplasty versus eye drops for first-line treatment of ocular hypertension and glaucoma (LiGHT): a multicentre randomised controlled trial. Lancet. 2019;393(10180):1505–16.
11. Traverso CE, Walt JG, Kelly SP, Hommer AH, Bron AM, Denis P, Nordmann JP, Renard JP, Bayer A, Grehn F, Pfeiffer N, Cedrone C, Gandolfi S, Orzalesi N, Nucci C, Rossetti L, Azuara-Blanco A, Bagnis A, Hitchings R, Salmon JF, Bricola G, Buchholz PM, Kotak SV, Katz LM, Siegartel LR, Doyle JJ. Direct costs of glaucoma and severity of the disease: a multinational long term study of resource utilisation in Europe. Br J Ophthalmol. 2005;89(10):1245–9.
12. Sleath B, Blalock S, Covert D, Stone JL, Skinner AC, Muir K, Robin AL. The relationship between glaucoma medication adherence, eye drop technique, and visual field defect severity. Ophthalmology. 2011;118(12):2398–402.
13. Zhou J, Smedley GT. A trabecular bypass flow hypothesis. J Glaucoma. 2005;14(1):74–83.
14. Rosenquist R, Epstein D, Melamed S, Johnson M, Grant WM. Outflow resistance of enucleated human eyes at two different perfusion pressures and different extents of trabeculotomy. Curr Eye Res. 1989;8(12):1233–40.
15. Grover DS, Smith O, Fellman RL, Godfrey DG, Gupta A, Montes de Oca I, Feuer WJ. Gonioscopy-assisted transluminal trabeculotomy: an ab interno circumferential trabeculotomy: 24 months follow-up. J Glaucoma. 2018;27(5):393–401.
16. Rahmatnejad K, Pruzan NL, Amanullah S, Shaukat BA, Resende AF, Waisbourd M, Zhan T, Moster MR. Surgical outcomes of Gonioscopy-assisted Transluminal Trabeculotomy (GATT) in patients with open-angle glaucoma. J Glaucoma. 2017;26(12):1137–43.
17. Baykara M, Poroy C, Erseven C. Surgical outcomes of combined gonioscopy-assisted transluminal trabeculotomy and cataract surgery. Indian J Ophthalmol. 2019;67(4):505–8.
18. Minckler D, Mosaed S, Dustin L, Brian Francis M, Trabectome Study Group. Trabectome (trabeculectomy-internal approach): additional experience and extended follow-up. Trans Am Ophthalmol Soc. 2008;106:149–59. discussion 159–60
19. Ting JL, Damji KF, Stiles MC, Trabectome Study Group. Ab interno trabeculectomy: outcomes in exfoliation versus primary open-angle glaucoma. J Cataract Refract Surg. 2012;38(2):315–23.

20. Ahuja Y, Ma Khin Pyi S, Malihi M, Hodge DO, Sit AJ. Clinical results of ab interno trabeculotomy using the trabectome for open-angle glaucoma: the Mayo Clinic series in Rochester, Minnesota. Am J Ophthalmol. 2013;156(5):927–935.e2.
21. Dorairaj SK, Kahook MY, Williamson BK, Seibold LK, ElMallah MK, Singh IP. A multicenter retrospective comparison of goniotomy versus trabecular bypass device implantation in glaucoma patients undergoing cataract extraction. Clin Ophthalmol. 2018;12:791–7.
22. Berdahl JP, Gallardo MJ, ElMallah MK, Williamson BK, Kahook MY, Mahootchi A, Rappaport LA, Lazcano-Gomez GS, Díaz-Robles D, Dorairaj SK. Six-month outcomes of goniotomy performed with the Kahook dual blade as a stand-alone glaucoma procedure. Adv Ther. 2018;35(11):2093–102.
23. Salinas L, Chaudhary A, Berdahl JP, Lazcano-Gomez GS, Williamson BK, Dorairaj SK, Seibold LK, Smith S, Aref AA, Darlington JK, Jimenez-Roman J, Mahootchi A, Boucekine M, Mansouri K. Goniotomy using the Kahook dual blade in severe and refractory glaucoma: 6-month outcomes. J Glaucoma. 2018;27(10):849–55.
24. Gallardo MJ, Supnet RA, Ahmed IIK. Viscodilation of Schlemm's canal for the reduction of IOP via an ab-interno approach. Clin Ophthalmol. 2018;12:2149–55.
25. Battista SA, Lu Z, Hofmann S, Freddo TF, Overby DR, Gong H. Reduction of the available area for aqueous humor outflow and increase in meshwork herniations into collector channels following acute IOP elevation in bovine eyes. Invest Ophthalmol Vis Sci. 2008;49:5346–52.
26. Lewis RA, von Wolff K, Tetz M, Koerber N, Kearney JR, Shingleton BJ, Samuelson TW. Canaloplasty: three-year results of circumferential viscodilation and tensioning of Schlemm's canal using a microcatheter to treat open-angle glaucoma. J Cataract Refract Surg. 2011;37:682–90.
27. Ahmed IIK, Fea A, Au L, Ang RE, Harasymowycz P, Jampel H, Samuelson TW, Chang DF, Rhee DJ, COMPARE Investigators. A prospective randomized trial comparing Hydrus and iStent micro-invasive glaucoma glaucoma surgery implants for standalone treatment of open-angle glaucoma: The COMPARE Study. Ophthalmology. 2019;S0161-6420:31710-X.
28. Katz LJ, Erb C, Carceller Guillamet A, Fea AM, Voskanyan L, Wells JM, Giamporcaro JE. Prospective, randomized study of one, two, or three trabecular bypass stents in openangle glaucoma subjects on topical hypotensive medication. Clin Ophthalmol. 2015;9:2313–20.
29. Fea AM, Belda JI, Rękas M, Jünemann A, Chang L, Pablo L, Voskanyan L, Katz LJ. Prospective unmasked randomized evaluation of the istent inject versus two ocular hypotensive agents in patients with primary open-angle glaucoma. Clin Ophthalmol. 2014;8:875–82.
30. Fea AM, Ahmed II, Lavia C, Mittica P, Consolandi G, Motolese I, Pignata G, Motolese E, Rolle T, Frezzotti P. Hydrus microstent compared to selective laser trabeculoplasty in primary open angle glaucoma: one year results. Clin Exp Ophthalmol. 2017;45:120–7.
31. Preliminary ASCRS CyPass withdrawal consensus statement. ASCRS. 2018. http://ascrs.org/CyPass_Statement. Accessed 19 May 2019.
32. Durr G, Ahmed IIK. Endothelial cell loss and MIGS: what we know and don't know. Glaucoma Today. September/October 2018. http://glaucomatoday.com/2018/10/endothelial-cell-loss-and-migs-what-we-know-and-dont-know/
33. Lee EK, Yun YJ, Lee JE, Yim JH, Kim CS. Changes in corneal endothelial cells after Ahmed glaucoma valve implantation: 2-year follow-up. Am J Ophthalmol. 2009;148(3):361–7.
34. Kim KN, Lee SB, Lee YH, Lee JJ, Lim HB, Kim CS. Changes in corneal endothelial cell density and the cumulative risk of corneal decompensation after Ahmed glaucoma valve implantation. Br J Ophthalmol. 2016;100(7):933–8.
35. Tan AN, Webers CA, Berendschot TT, et al. Corneal endothelial cell loss after Baerveldt glaucoma drainage device implantation in the anterior chamber. Acta Ophthalmol. 2017;95(1):91–6.
36. Tojo N, Hayashi A, Consolvo-Ueda T, Yanagisawa S. Baerveldt surgery outcomes: anterior chamber insertion versus vitreous cavity insertion. Graefes Arch Clin Exp Ophthalmol. 2018;6:2191–200. https://doi.org/10.1007/s00417-018-4116-4.
37. Arnavielle S, Lafontaine PO, Bidot S, Creuzot-Garcher C, D'Athis P, Bron AM. Corneal endothelial cell changes after trabeculectomy and deep sclerectomy. J Glaucoma. 2007;16(3):324–8.
38. Nassiri N, Nassiri N, Rahnavardi M, Rahmani L. A comparison of corneal endothelial cell changes after 1-site and 2-site phacotrabeculectomy. Cornea. 2008;27(8):889–94.

39. Storr-Paulsen T, Norregaard JC, Ahmed S, Storr-Paulsen A. Corneal endothelial cell loss after mitomycin C-augmented trabeculectomy. J Glaucoma. 2008;17(8):654–7.
40. Konopińska J, Deniziak M, Saeed E, et al. Prospective randomized study comparing combined phaco-ExPress and phacotrabeculectomy in open angle glaucoma treatment: 12-month follow-up. J Ophthalmol. 2015;2015:720109.
41. Buys YM, Chipman ML, Zack B, Rootman DS, Slomovic AR, Trope GE. Prospective randomized comparison of one- versus two-site phacotrabeculectomy two-year results. Ophthalmology. 2008;115(7):1130–1133.e1.
42. Samuelson TW, Chang DF, Marquis R, HORIZON Investigators, et al. A Schlemm canal microstent for intraocular pressure reduction in primary open-angle glaucoma and cataract: the HORIZON study. Ophthalmology. 126:29–37. https://doi.org/10.1016/j.ophtha.2018.05.012.
43. Arriola-Villalobos P, Martínez-de-la-Casa JM, et al. Mid-term evaluation of the new Glaukos iStent with phacoemulsification in coexistent open-angle glaucoma or ocular hypertension and cataract. Br J Ophthalmol. 2013;97(10):1250–5.
44. Maeda M, Watanabe M, Ichikawa K. Evaluation of trabectome in open-angle glaucoma. J Glaucoma. 2013;22(3):205–8.
45. Fea AM, Spinetta R, Cannizzo PML, et al. Evaluation of bleb morphology and reduction in IOP and glaucoma medication following implantation of a novel gel stent. J Ophthalmol. 2017;2017:9364910.
46. Row H. Operation to control glaucoma. Arch Ophthalmol. 1935;12:325–9.
47. Alm A, Nilsson SF. Uveoscleral outflow—a review. Exp Eye Res. 2009;88(4):760–8.
48. Samples JR, Ahmed IIK. Surgical innovations in glaucoma. 1st ed. New York: Springer Science. p. 33–41.
49. Troncoso MU. Cyclodialysis with insertion of a metal implant in the treatment of glaucoma. Arch Ophthalmol. 1940;23:270–300.
50. Bick MW. Use of tantalum for ocular drainage. Arch Ophthalmol. 1949;42:375–88.
51. Bietti GB. The present state of the use of plastics in eye surgery. Acta Ophthalmol. 1955;33:337–70.
52. Klemm M, Balazs A, Draeger J, Wiezorrek R. Experimental use of space-retaining substances with extended duration: functional and morphological results. Graefes Arch Clin Exp Ophthalmol. 1995;233(9):592–7.
53. Jordan JF, Engels BF, Dinslage S, et al. A novel approach to suprachoroidal drainage for the surgical treatment of intractable glaucoma. J Glaucoma. 2006;15(3):200–5.
54. Melamed S, Ben Simon GJ, Goldenfeld M, Simon G. Efficacy and safety of gold micro shunt implantation to the supraciliary space in patients with glaucoma: a pilot study. Arch Ophthalmol. 2009;127(3):264–9.
55. Fili S, Wölfelschneider P, Kohlhaas M. The STARflo glaucoma implant: preliminary 12 months results. Graefes Arch Clin Exp Ophthalmol. 2018;256(4):773–81.
56. Potential eye damage from Alcon CyPass Micro-Stent used to treat open-angle glaucoma: FDA safety communication. FDA. September 14, 2018. www.fda.gov/MedicalDevices/Safety/AlertsandNotices/ucm620646.htm.
57. Endothelial cell loss and MIGS: what we know and don't know. September–October 2018. http://glaucomatoday.com/2018/10/endothelial-cell-loss-and-migs-what-we-know-and-dont-know/
58. Hopen ML, Patel S, Gallardo MJ. Cypass supraciliary stent in eye with chronic angle closure and postvitrectomy with silicone oil. J Glaucoma. 2018;27(10):e151–3.
59. Myers JS, Masood I, Hornbeak DM, Belda JI, Auffarth G, Jünemann A, Giamporcaro JE, Martinez-de-la-Casa JM, Ahmed IIK, Voskanyan L, Katz LJ. Prospective evaluation of two iStent(®) trabecular stents, one iStent supra(®) suprachoroidal stent, and postoperative prostaglandin in refractory glaucoma: 4-year outcomes. Adv Ther. 2018;35(3):395–407.
60. Denis P, Hirneiß C, Reddy KP, Kamarthy A, Calvo E, Hussain Z, Ahmed IIK. A first-in-human study of the efficacy and safety of MINIject in patients with medically uncontrolled open-angle glaucoma (STAR-I). Ophthalmol Glaucoma. 2019;2:290–7. https://doi.org/10.1016/j.ogla.2019.06.001.

61. Gedde SJ, Schiffman JC, Feuer WJ, Herndon LW, Brandt JD, Budenz DL. Treatment outcomes in the tube versus trabeculectomy (TVT) study after five years of follow-up. Am J Ophthalmol. 2012;153(5):789–803.e2. https://doi.org/10.1016/j.ajo.2011.10.026.
62. Matlach J, Dhillon C, Hain J, Schlunck G, Grehn F, Klink T. Trabeculectomy versus canaloplasty (TVC study) in the treatment of patients with open-angle glaucoma: a prospective randomized clinical trial. Acta Ophthalmol. 2015;93:753–61. https://doi.org/10.1111/aos.12722.
63. Gedde SJ, Chen PP, Heuer DK, et al. The primary tube versus trabeculectomy study. Ophthalmology. 2018;125(5):774–81. https://doi.org/10.1016/j.ophtha.2017.10.037.
64. Gedde SJ, Feuer WJ, Shi W, et al. Treatment outcomes in the primary tube versus trabeculectomy study after 1 year of follow-up. Ophthalmology. 2018;125(5):650–63. https://doi.org/10.1016/j.ophtha.2018.02.003.
65. Kirwan JF, Lockwood AJ, Shah P, et al. Trabeculectomy in the 21st century: a multicenter analysis. Ophthalmology. 2013;120:2532–9. https://doi.org/10.1016/j.ophtha.2013.07.049.
66. Reitsamer H, Sng C, Vera V, et al. Two-year results of a multicenter study of the ab interno gelatin implant in medically uncontrolled primary open-angle glaucoma. Graefes Arch Clin Exp Ophthalmol. 2019;257:983–96. https://doi.org/10.1007/s00417-019-04251-z.
67. Schlenker MB, Gulamhusein H, Conrad-Hengerer I, et al. Efficacy, safety, and risk factors for failure of standalone Ab Interno Gelatin microstent implantation versus standalone trabeculectomy. Ophthalmology. 2017;124:1579–88. https://doi.org/10.1016/j.ophtha.2017.05.004.
68. Pinchuk L, Wilson GJ, Barry JJ, Schoephoerster RT, Parel JM, Kennedy JP. Medical applications of poly(styrene-block-isobutylene-block-styrene) ("SIBS"). Biomaterials. 2008;29(60):448. https://doi.org/10.1016/j.biomaterials.2007.09.041.
69. Batlle JF, Fantes F, Riss I, et al. Three-year follow-up of a novel aqueous humor microshunt. J Glaucoma. 2016;25:e58–65. https://doi.org/10.1097/IJG.0000000000000368.

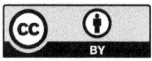

Globalization of MIGS

11

Chelvin C. A. Sng, Clement C. Tham, Donald L. Budenz, Paul R. Healey, and Ningli Wang

11.1   Introduction

Good health for all populations is an accepted international goal. Globalization is the process of interaction and integration among people, companies, and governments worldwide and was previously regarded as a predominantly economic process. However, it is increasingly perceived as a more comprehensive phenomenon with significant implications for global health. The relationship between globalization and health is complex and globalization is a multifaceted phenomenon which can influence health in a myriad of ways. Globalization facilitates the spread of modern medicine and medical devices, extending life expectancy in developing countries from 55 years in 1970 to 65 years in 1997. However, it can also exacerbate the gap between the rich and the poor, both among and within countries.

C. C. A. Sng (✉)
Department of Ophthalmology, National University Hospital, Singapore, Singapore

Singapore Eye Research Institute, Singapore, Singapore

C. C. Tham
Department of Ophthalmology and Visual Sciences, The Chinese University of Hong Kong, Shatin, New Territories, Hong Kong SAR

Hong Kong Eye Hospital, Kowloon, Hong Kong SAR

D. L. Budenz
Department of Ophthalmology, School of Medicine, University of North Carolina at Chapel Hill, Chapel Hill, NC, USA

P. R. Healey
Centre for Vision Research, Westmead Institute for Medical Research, University of Sydney, Sydney, NSW, Australia

N. Wang
Beijing Tongren Eye Center, Beijing Tongren Hospital, Capital Medical University, Beijing Ophthalmology and Visual Science Key Laboratory, Beijing, China

© The Author(s) 2021   147
C. C. A. Sng, K. Barton (eds.), *Minimally Invasive Glaucoma Surgery*,
https://doi.org/10.1007/978-981-15-5632-6_11

While knowledge of and interest in minimally invasive glaucoma surgery (MIGS) has spread across the globe, access is far from global. Prior to 2016, MIGS devices were available mainly in Europe and Canada, with the exception of the iStent trabecular micro-bypass stent, which was also commercialized in the United States and selected countries in Asia (Singapore and Hong Kong). Since 2016, the US Food and Drug Administration (FDA) has approved the CyPass Micro-Stent (Alcon Laboratories Inc., Fort Worth, Tx USA) (August 2016, subsequently withdrawn in August 2018), the XEN Gel Implant (Allergan plc, Dublin, Ireland) (November 2016), the iStent Inject (Glaukos Corporation, San Clemente, CA, USA) (June 2018), and the Hydrus Microstent (Ivantis Inc., Irvine, CA, USA) (August 2018). These devices are also slowly making inroads into Asia, Australasia, South America, and South Africa.

The global prevalence of glaucoma is anticipated to increase from 64.3 million in 2013 to 111.8 million in 2040, disproportionately affecting people in Asia and Africa [1]. MIGS companies may foresee a quantum leap in economies of scale by serving global markets rather than only a confined domestic market.

11.2 Cost

In view of the costly commercialization process and the expensive acquisitions of several MIGS start-ups by multinational companies, MIGS devices are currently priced at a premium. For instance, the price of the XEN Gel Implant has more than doubled in Europe since Aquesys was acquired by Allergan in 2015. Hence, the go-to-market strategy for most MIGS companies has focused on countries where a significant proportion of healthcare coverage is provided through private health insurance (e.g., United States and Australia) or public health funding (e.g., the United Kingdom and Canada). The latter often requires the technology to be appraised and recommended by certain national institutes based on clinical and economic evidence. For instance, the National Institute for Health and Care Excellence (NICE) in the United Kingdom carries out periodic health technology assessments of new entrants. While not legally binding, a NICE assessment carries a great deal of weight for or against the adoption of new technology.

Some studies have reported MIGS cost-effectiveness in such reimbursement environments. In the Canadian healthcare setting, Patel et al. projected that two iStent Trabecular Micro-Bypass Stents were cost-effective compared with standard-of-care treatment with glaucoma medication in patients with mild-to-moderate open-angle glaucoma for more than 15 years, with quality-of-life gains [2]. Ngan et al. compared iStent accompanying cataract surgery with topical glaucoma medication in a public healthcare setting in New Zealand and found that the iStent is reasonably cost-effective, particularly for those using more expensive topical glaucoma medications [3]. Indeed, the cost-effectiveness of MIGS procedures may vary depending on whether brand name or generic eye drops are used. In the Manchester iStent study, Tan and Au found that the overall cost of combined cataract surgery and iStent implantation was GBP£7.70 per patient per year more than conservative management with brand name eyedrops, but GBP£131.3 per patient per year more if generic eyedrops were used [4]. Nevertheless, a systematic literature review of clinical and economic outcomes of MIGS in primary open-angle glaucoma highlighted that the available evidence on the cost-effectiveness of MIGS is limited and it remains unclear whether the cost of using MIGS is outweighed by cost savings through decreased medication and need for further interventions [5]. The price–performance ratio of MIGS is also an important consideration. The Microcatheter (iTrack 250A, iScience Interventional, Menlo Park, CA, USA) and Trabectome (NeoMedix Corporation, San Juan Capistrano, CA, USA) are available in the Chinese market, but these procedures are expensive and the surgical expenses are not covered by basic medical insurance. Hence, they are not widely performed in China. Evidently, there is still significant room for growth in the large Chinese glaucoma surgical market.

Ultimately, the global scalability of MIGS would be more dependent on cost and ease of implantation than efficacy. Unfortunately, out-of-pocket payments constitute a significant part of the health financing landscape in many countries. While MIGS may still be affordable in the wealthier of such countries (e.g., Singapore and Hong Kong), the cost of these devices is prohibitive for a significant proportion of the world's population, especially in Asia and Africa. In these large albeit cost-sensitive markets, the cheapest MIGS device is likely to prevail and outperform its competitors. In particular, current treatment options for glaucoma patients in developing countries remain limited and unsustainable. Even if these patients are diagnosed at an early stage of the disease, their prognosis remains dire. The recurrent cost of glaucoma medication renders them unaffordable in the long run. The lack of patient understanding of their disease results in poor compliance with medication and conventional glaucoma surgery (i.e., trabeculectomy) is often not feasible due to the difficulty of postoperative care, unpredictable results, and possible surgical complications. New glaucoma surgical treatment options, for example MIGS, that are safer and require less postoperative management, are particularly promising in this context. Ordonez et al. projected that the iStent Trabecular Micro-Bypass Stent would be a highly cost-saving procedure in the Colombian healthcare system due to more quality-adjusted life-years related to a lower rate of the population with loss of visual acuity in the long term [6]. Despite being potentially vision-saving, the cost of these new innovations prohibits their use in developing countries where they are most needed and the potential surgical volumes are the highest. Reducing the price of these devices in exchange for an increase in sales volume will chart a more profitable path in these resource-poor markets.

11.3   Distribution Channels

After Glaukos Corporation, which developed the iStent Trabecular Micro-Bypass Stent, staged a hugely successful initial public offering (IPO) in June 2015, the MIGS world has been rocked by a series of high-profile and multimillion dollar acquisitions. Allergan purchased Aquesys and its XEN Gel Implant with a US$325 million upfront payment in the third quarter of 2015. This was followed by the similarly expensive acquisitions of Transcend Medical and its CyPass Micro-Stent by

Alcon (withdrawn in August 2018) and the InnFocus MicroShunt (now renamed PRESERFLO MicroShunt) by Santen in 2016. With these developments, the MIGS landscape has evolved rapidly from a medley of start-ups to a battleground of industry heavyweights.

The acquisition of MIGS devices by multinational pharmaceutical and biotechnology companies, which have established international distribution channels, will undeniably facilitate the globalization of MIGS. In contrast, the smaller MIGS companies that have not been acquired often have to rely on local distributors to access international markets and have to be more selective with their target markets. There are certainly opportunities for mutually beneficial partnerships to be forged between the MIGS companies in their quest for global expansion. An illustrative example is a multi-year agreement between Glaukos and Santen whereby Glaukos will become the exclusive distributor of the MicroShunt solely in the US market once it is approved by the FDA. This will allow Santen to concentrate on the European and Asian markets while leveraging on Glaukos's established distribution and sales infrastructure in the United States.

11.4   Surgical Training

A major constraint in the globalization of MIGS is the limited resources available for surgeon training and education. The inadequate availability of surgical trainers (who may require years of experience before reaching competence) and real patients for supervised surgery creates a bottleneck in the training of MIGS surgeons. In addition, the number of free training devices provided by MIGS manufacturers is often insufficient for surgeons to overcome their learning curve. To address these deficiencies and to prevent them from compromising training standards, an expanded role for augmented and virtual reality in MIGS surgical training should be explored [7]. Virtual reality-based simulators for MIGS surgery may be able to reduce the learning curve, improve the conceptual understanding of ocular anatomy and enhance visuospatial skills, augmenting (albeit not replacing) the guidance provided by surgical trainers. Improvements in information technology have also dramatically increased the speed and ease of data flow, facilitating the sharing of information. To rapidly disseminate didactic training material on MIGS, such resources should be made freely available online in various languages. However, surgeons should be advised to access such information only through reputable websites and sources, so as to prevent the potentially rapid dissemination of misinformation. For instance, www.migs.org is a noncommercial site offering patient information leaflets in multiple languages. The Asia-Pacific Glaucoma Society has established a MIGS Interest Group and developed patient information leaflets for MIGS devices which are available online (www.apglaucomasociety.org/migs) (Fig. 11.1). Other international and regional glaucoma societies may consider similar initiatives to improve surgeon and patient education. It is imperative that surgical standards are not compromised in the process of globalization, to ensure consistently good outcomes from MIGS.

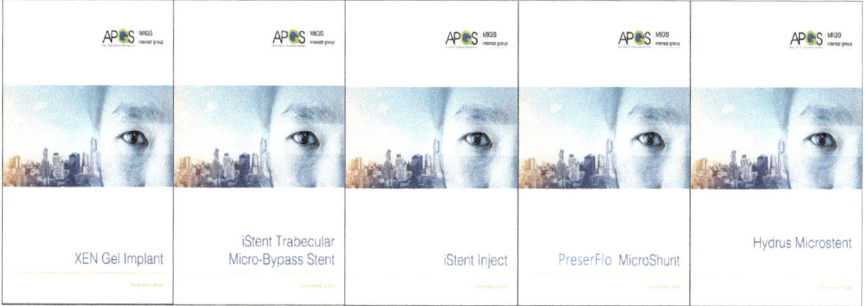

Fig. 11.1 Asia-Pacific Glaucoma Society patient information leaflets for minimally invasive glaucoma surgery devices which are available at www.apglaucomasociety.org/migs. (Image provided by Chelvin Sng, FRCSEd)

Fig. 11.2 Anterior segment photograph of a diffuse bleb associated with the XEN Gel Implant in a Chinese eye with thick Tenon's capsule, showing that the implant is not visible when it is located under the Tenon's capsule. (Copyright Chelvin Sng, FRCSEd; reproduced with permission)

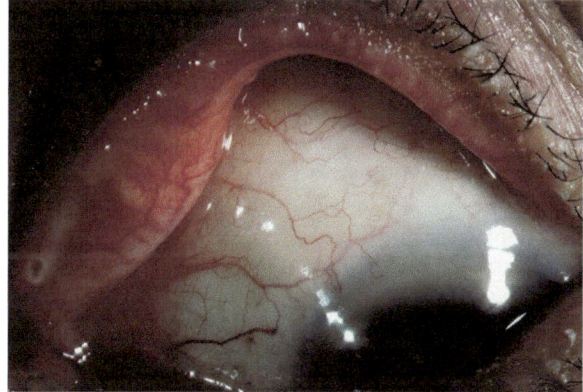

11.5 Patients

Currently, the published data on MIGS procedures mostly pertain to Caucasian eyes and it remains uncertain whether these devices will be just as effective in Asian or African eyes. This is especially relevant for the subconjunctival MIGS devices, as Asian and African eyes have a propensity for subconjunctival scarring [8, 9]. The Tenon's capsule is also significantly thicker in African and Asian eyes compared with Caucasian eyes, which may predispose to the occlusion of subconjunctival MIGS devices. For instance, the XEN Gel Implant is an ab-interno subconjunctival MIGS device that is typically implanted without a conjunctival peritomy, but in some African and Asian eyes with very thick Tenon's (Fig. 11.2), it may be necessary to perform a conjunctival peritomy to ensure proper placement of the implant (Fig. 11.3). It may also be necessary to apply a higher concentration of antimetabolites intraoperatively and to prescribe a longer duration of postoperative topical

Fig. 11.3 Implantation of the XEN Gel Implant with conjunctival peritomy. (Copyright Chelvin Sng, FRCSEd; reproduced with permission)

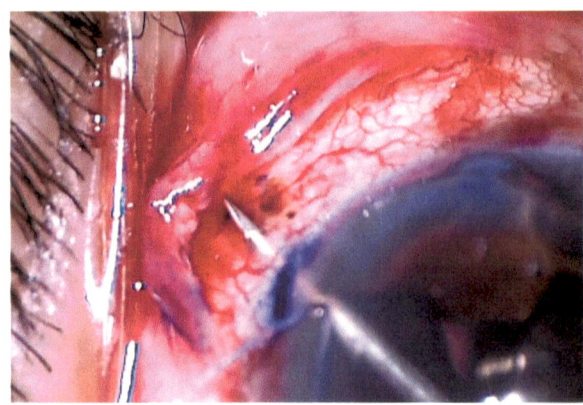

steroids for subconjunctival MIGS devices to achieve similar rates of surgical success as that in Caucasian eyes, although further studies are required to verify these hypotheses.

Despite the size of the Chinese market, with a high prevalence of glaucoma, the availability of MIGS and other novel glaucoma surgical options is currently very limited. One exception is the Microcatheter (iTrack 250A, iScience Interventional, Menlo Park, CA, USA), which was introduced in China in 2012 by Wang's team. This typically requires a conjunctival peritomy and the creation of a scleral flap and is not considered minimally invasive. Wang's team subsequently simplified the canaloplasty surgical procedure in China to introduce *reconstruction of aqueous outflow drainage (RAOD)* surgery, omitting two steps (creation of the scleral lake and Descemet's membrane window). This simplified procedure has been used to treat eyes with multiple failed glaucoma filtration procedures and disrupted Schlemm's canal observed by gonioscopy (relay technique) [10]. They also pioneered the use of partial circumferential trabeculotomy with the Microcatheter in primary congenital glaucoma after failed angle surgeries, which may achieve similar postoperative IOP as 360° trabeculotomy. Refractory glaucoma with previous failed conventional glaucoma filtration procedures is a significant challenge in China and bleb-less surgery may be a viable surgical option for these eyes, although the postoperative IOP may not be low enough for advanced glaucoma. The Trabectome is also available in China and has been shown to be effective and safe in a multicenter retrospective study [11]. With the introduction of such new surgical options, trabeculectomy rates in China have gradually declined. The surgical outcomes of other MIGS procedures in Chinese eyes still require investigation.

Data on MIGS outcomes in glaucoma subtypes besides primary open-angle glaucoma are limited. The efficacy of MIGS in certain subtypes of glaucoma, such as angle-closure glaucoma which is prevalent in Asia, would need to be established. In an exploratory, prospective, interventional case series, Hernstadt et al. showed that combined iStent trabecular micro-bypass stent insertion and phacoemulsification was effective in lowering the intraocular pressure (14.8 ± 3.9 vs. 17.5 ± 3.8 mmHg at baseline; $p = 0.008$) and the number of glaucoma medications (0.14 ± 0.48 vs.

1.49 ± 0.77 at baseline; $p < 0.001$) for at least 12 months, with a favorable safety profile. Despite cataract extraction, postoperative iStent occlusion with iris occurred in 27.0% of the eyes, which is much higher than the incidence of stent occlusion reported after iStent implantation in eyes with open-angle glaucoma (4–18%) [12]. In a prospective, single-masked, randomized study comparing the efficacy of combined phacoemulsification and iStent implantation with standard phacoemulsification in eyes with primary angle closure disease, the combined surgery was associated with a higher likelihood of complete success at 12 months (87.5% [95% CI 58.6–96.7 vs 43.8% [95% CI 19.8–65.6]; $p = 0.01$) [13]. Sng et al. reported that combined XEN implantation with cataract surgery was effective in lowering IOP and the number of glaucoma medications in 31 Chinese eyes with primary open-angle glaucoma and primary angle-closure glaucoma for at least 12 months, with a favorable safety profile [14]. However, implant occlusion with iris may occur more frequently in angle-closure eyes, even after cataract surgery (Fig. 11.4). This exploratory study was unable to distinguish between the IOP-lowering effect of XEN and phacoemulsification and more randomized controlled studies comparing combined phacoemulsification with MIGS and phacoemulsification alone are required.

Trabecular bypass procedures and newer modalities of cycloablation are attractive surgical options for patients in less developed nations as they do not require much postoperative management or medications. However, cycloablative procedures may increase conjunctival scarring and compromise the success of subsequent

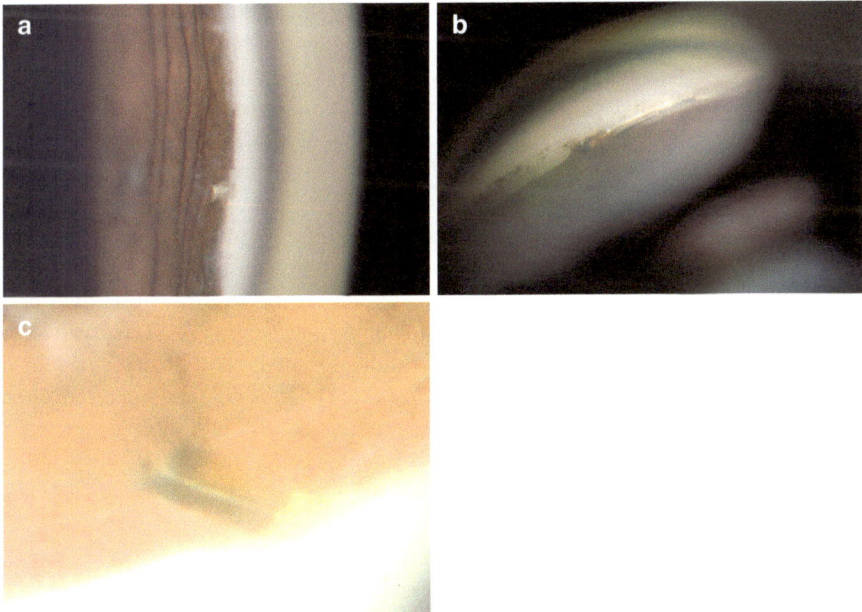

Fig. 11.4 Gonioscopy photographs showing iris occlusion of the (**a**) iStent Trabecular Micro-Bypass Stent, the (**b**) Hydrus Microstent, and the (**c**) XEN Gel Implant in angle-closure glaucoma eyes even after cataract extraction. (Copyright Chelvin Sng, FRCSEd; reproduced with permission)

conjunctival filtration surgery [15]. Trabecular bypass procedures have a high safety profile and spare the conjunctiva, but the modest efficacy of these procedures renders them more appropriate for patients with the mild-to-moderate disease who would otherwise be noncompliant with their glaucoma medications. In reality, due to the poor access to healthcare and eye screening programs, a significant number of patients in less developed nations present with advanced glaucoma. Subconjunctival MIGS devices, such as the InnFocus Microshunt (renamed PRESERFLO MicroShunt), are more likely to achieve lower target IOP compared with other MIGS devices, with a lower rate of complications compared with trabeculectomy [16], but require postoperative bleb management and possibly a longer duration of topical steroids. There is currently an unmet need for a MIGS device that requires minimal postoperative management and yet is able to reduce IOP sufficiently for patients with advanced glaucoma.

11.6   Regulatory Considerations and Other Concerns

Regulatory restrictions remain a roadblock for the globalization of MIGS. It is important for MIGS manufacturers to understand the legal and regulatory climate before entering a new market. Such information is vital for strategic decisions about where and how to expand globally. Countries with fewer regulatory barriers (e.g., Europe, Canada, and Singapore) often have earlier access to MIGS devices. On the other hand, certain countries (e.g., United States and China) have more stringent requirements. The US-FDA's strict adherence to evidence-based evaluation of medical devices often results in a notoriously drawn-out and bureaucratic approval process. The Chinese FDA (CFDA) requirement for data from Chinese patients is similarly challenging. When submitting international multicenter clinical trial data for CFDA evaluation, the overseas applicant is obliged to show that the enrolled Chinese trial subjects are representative of the relevant patient population in Chinese medical practice and that the sample size of Chinese subjects meets statistical requirements. As it may be daunting to conduct a clinical trial in China, a feasible alternative would be to obtain supplementary data from other countries with predominantly Chinese populations (e.g., Singapore and Hong Kong). Nevertheless, the United States and China are two of the largest markets globally and remain coveted despite their regulatory difficulties. While most MIGS manufacturers target the US market after establishing their devices in Europe, a notable exception is EyeTechCare (manufacturer of High-Intensity Focused Ultrasound [EyeOP1 HIFU, EyeTechCare, Rillieux-la-Pape, France]), which received CFDA approval for its device ahead of US-FDA approval. This alternative commercialization strategy affords the company the first-mover advantage in a large and untapped Chinese market, although the long-term advantages of this strategy are yet to be established.

Another consideration in the globalization of MIGS is the protection of intellectual property, which remains a concern in lesser-developed countries despite the Agreement on Trade-Related Aspects of Intellectual Property Rights (1994). Indeed, it may be difficult to seek legal recourse for intellectual property infringements in certain countries, and under such circumstances, the value of novel biomaterials or trade secrets may exceed that of patents in intellectual property protection.

11.7 Conclusion

The path to MIGS globalization is fraught with adversity as well as opportunity. Despite the economic, logistic, training, legal and regulatory challenges discussed earlier, the permeation of MIGS devices internationally is an inevitable reality. Ultimately, the success of these devices in the global market will distinguish the survivors from the casualties. It is anticipated that the health benefits of globalization will outweigh the disadvantages, and glaucoma patients worldwide stand to gain from increased access to MIGS devices, which might reduce glaucoma medication burden and improve quality of life. Whether such new technology can decrease the global incidence of glaucoma-related blindness remains to be seen, but this is certainly a worthy aspiration.

References

1. Quigley HA. Number of people with glaucoma worldwide. Br J Ophthalmol. 1996;80:389–93.
2. Patel V, Ahmed I, Podbielski D, Falvey H, Murray J, Goeree R. Cost-effectiveness analysis of standalone trabecular micro-bypass stents in patients with mild-to-moderate open-angle glaucoma in Canada. J Med Econ. 2019;22:390–401.
3. Ngan K, Fraser E, Buller S, Buller A. A cost minimisation analysis comparing iStent accompanying cataract surgery and selective laser trabeculoplasty versus topical glaucoma medications in a public healthcare setting in New Zealand. Graefes Arch Clin Exp Ophthalmol. 2018;256:2181–9.
4. Tan SZ, Au L. Manchester iStent study: 3-year results and cost analysis. Eye (Lond). 2016;30:1365–70.
5. Agrawal P, Bradshaw SE. Systematic literature review of clinical and economic outcomes of micro-invasive glaucoma surgery (MIGS) in primary open-angle glaucoma. Ophthalmol Ther. 2018;7:749–73.
6. Ordonez JE, Ordonez A, Osorio UM. Cost-effectiveness analysis of iStent trabecular micro-bypass stent for patients with open-angle glaucoma in Colombia. Curr Med Res Opin. 2019;35:329–40.
7. Jacobsen MF, Konge L, Bach-Holm D, et al. Correlation of virtual reality performance with real-life cataract surgery performance. J Cataract Refract Surg. 2019;45:1246–51. [Epub ahead of print]
8. Nguyen AH, Fatehi N, Romero P, et al. Observational outcomes of initial trabeculectomy with mitomycin C in patients of African descent vs patients of European descent: five-year results. JAMA Ophthalmol. 2018;136:1106–13.
9. Husain R, Clarke JC, Seah SK, Khaw PT. A review of trabeculectomy in East Asian people—the influence of race. Eye (Lond). 2005;19:243–52.
10. Xin C, Tian N, Li M, Wang H, Wang N. Mechanism of the reconstruction of aqueous outflow drainage. Sci China Life Sci. 2018;61:534–40.

11. Dang YL, Cen YJ, Hong Y, et al. Safety and efficacy of trabectome-mediated trabecular mesh-work ablation for Chinese glaucoma patients: a two-year, retrospective, multicentre study. Chin Med J. 2018;131:420–5.
12. Hernstadt DJ, Cheng J, Htoon HM, Sangtam T, Thomas A, Sng CCA. Case series of combined iStent implantation and phacoemulsification in eyes with primary angle closure disease: one-year outcomes. Adv Ther. 2019;36:976–86.
13. David Z, Chen, Chelvin CA. Sng, Tiakumzuk Sangtam, Anoop Thomas, Liang Shen, Philemon K. Huang, Jason Cheng. Phacoemulsification vs phacoemulsification with micro-bypass stent implantation in primary angle closure and primary angle closure glaucoma: A randomized single-masked clinical study. Clin Exp Ophthalmol. 2020;48:450–61.
14. Chelvin C. A. Sng, Paul T. K. Chew, Hla Myint Htoon, Katherine Lun, Preethi Jeyabal, Marcus Ang. Case Series of Combined XEN Implantation and Phacoemulsification in Chinese Eyes: One-Year Outcomes. Adv Ther. 2019;36:3519–529.
15. Nicholas Y. Q. Tan, Marcus Ang, Anita S. Y. Chan, Veluchamy A. Barathi, Clement C. Tham, Keith Barton, Chelvin C. A. Sng. Transscleral cyclophotocoagulation and its histological effects on the conjunctiva. Sci Rep. 2019;9.
16. Santen Pharmaceutical. Santen Announces Topline Data for DE-128 (MicroShunt) Demonstrating Reductions in IOP and Medication Use in Patients with Glaucoma. Press Release, 30 Aug 2019. https://eyewire.news/articles/santen-announces-topline-data-for-de-128-microshunt-demonstrating-reductions-in-iop-and-medication-use-in-patients-with-glau-coma/. Accessed 18 Sep 2019.

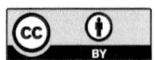

Appendix A: iStent Trabecular Micro-Bypass Stent Implantation Narrative Instructions

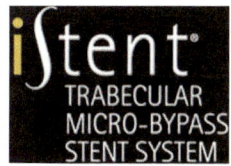

Step 1: Patient Positioning and Setup

To obtain proper viewing of the anterior chamber angle, turn the patient's head away from you (the surgeon) approximately 35° and turn the microscope toward you by approximately 35° (70° total). Position the gonioprism on the cornea to visualize the trabecular meshwork and ensure that a good view of the targeted implant site is available at the nasal implant location. To mitigate difficulty with patient movement or noncompliance, consider using a peri-bulbar or retrobulbar block.

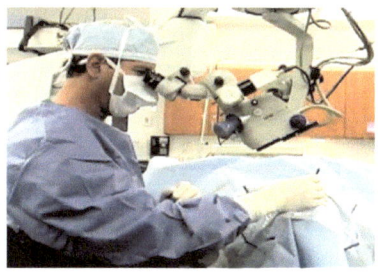

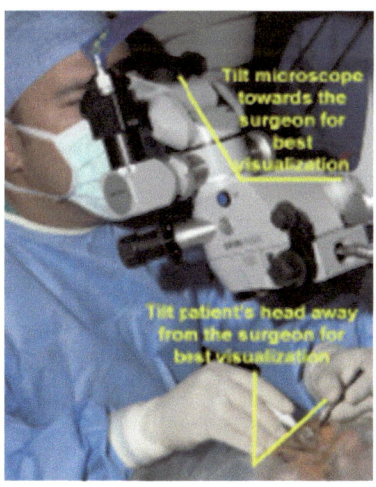

Step 2: Adjusting Microscope and Identifying Landmarks

Adjust the microscope setting to 10–12× and zoom and focus to locate the trabecular meshwork and identify the targeted stent implantation site. To visualize the targeted stent implantation location for the iStent Trabecular Micro-Bypass Stent® and the iStent *inject*®, focus on the landmarks shown in the image below and look anterior from the iris plane to find the scleral spur. The trabecular meshwork is located anterior to the scleral spur and is typically red/brown in color. Schlemm's canal is behind the trabecular meshwork.

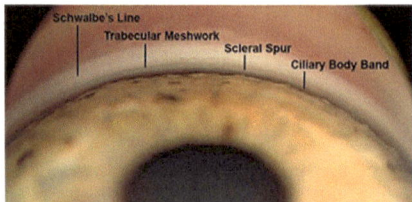 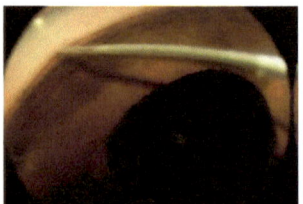

Step 3: Accessing Anterior Chamber

Deepen the anterior chamber with a cohesive viscoelastic as needed to maintain the chamber. When stent implantation is being performed with cataract surgery, enter the eye through the same corneal incision, otherwise create a 1.5 mm clear corneal incision for stent insertion. Prior to entering the eye, hold the inserter like a pencil, placing your index finger on the release button. Enter the corneal incision and guide the inserter across the pupillary margin (3–4 o'clock for the right eye; 8–9 o'clock for the left eye) and replace the gonioprism, taking care to avoid contact with the lens or cornea.

Step 4: Accessing Implantation Site

Locate the trabecular meshwork and select an implant location (shown below). Move the inserter to the left side (for the left eye) or right side (for the right eye) of the incision and engage the curvature of the trabecular meshwork with the tip of the stent, which has a self-trephining tip.

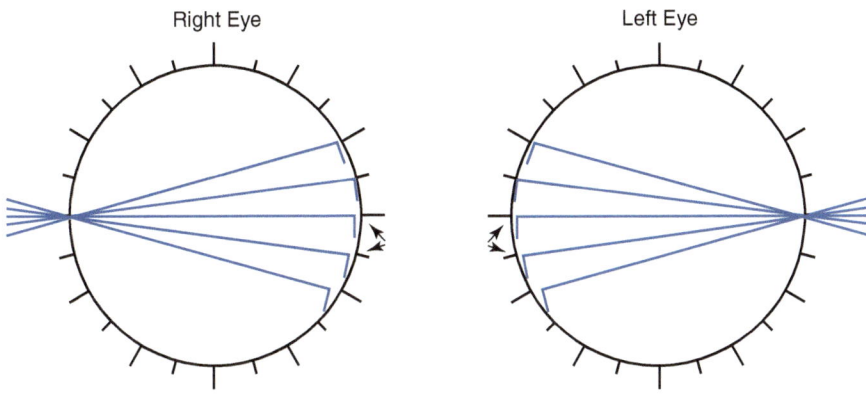

Implantation Approach Angle

Step 5: Stent Implantation (Left Eye Example)

Gently pierce the trabecular meshwork and advance the stent until the trabecular meshwork rides over the first retention arch. Plant the heel of the stent by moving the inserter to the opposite side of the incision. Slowly advance the stent to the left, engaging the tissue with the stent tip and sliding the stent under the trabecular meshwork and into the canal. Continue inserting until the iStent is fully advanced and the stent snorkel meets the trabecular meshwork.

If you encounter resistance or globe rotation, gently "tent" the trabecular meshwork tissue by pulling back toward the incision to create more space in the canal. When you are prepared to release the stent, slightly "dimple" into the trabecular meshwork (pushing toward the back wall of Schlemm's canal) and fully depress the inserter button to release the stent. Once the stent is in Schlemm's canal, gently tap the back of the snorkel with the inserter to fully seat the heel of the snorkel into the canal and confirm the stent placement by strumming the snorkel lightly up from below. Remove the inserter from the eye.

Before concluding the procedure, use gonioscopy to confirm correct placement. Minimal blood reflux is a normal physiological response to stent placement, although this does not occur in all cases.

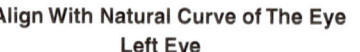

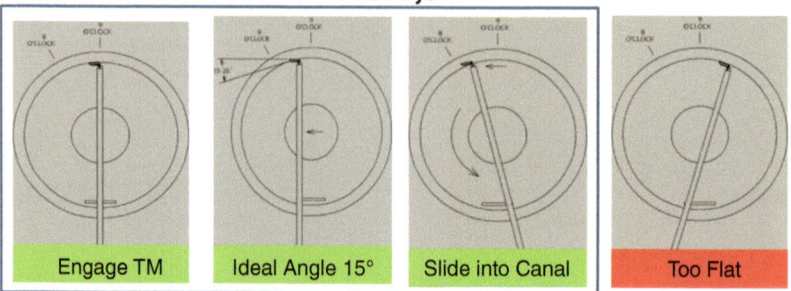

iStent Insertion Technique (Left eye – reverse for right eye):

1. Pass iStent across eye, remaining in center of corneal incision; engage trabecular meshwork (TM) at 15° angle.
2. Pass tip of iStent through TM into Schlemm's canal until tip encounters back wall of the canal. Inserter shaft should slide to left side of corneal incision.
3. Pull gently to lift TM and clear iStent tip from back wall of Schlemm's canal. Rotate inserter handle CCW toward right side of corneal incision. This will naturally advance iStent into the canal at the proper angle. Continue to slide until snorkel reaches TM incision.
4. Wrong location: If too flat or heel contacts with TM instead of tip, stent will not penetrate properly.

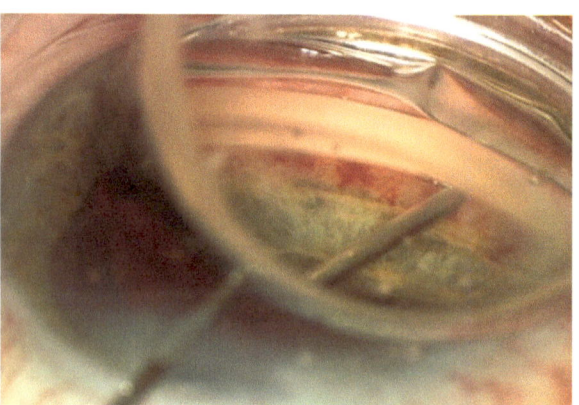

Step 6: Viscoelastic Removal

Using the corneal incision, irrigate and aspirate the anterior chamber with balanced salt solution (BSS) to remove all viscoelastic, pressing down on the posterior edge of the incision to facilitate complete removal of viscoelastic. Repeat as needed until all viscoelastic has been removed. Inflate the anterior chamber with saline solution to achieve physiologic pressure. Ensure that the corneal incision is sealed.

Appendix B: iStent *inject* Implantation Narrative Instructions

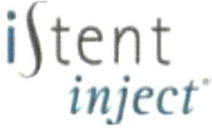

Step 1: Patient Positioning and Setup

To obtain proper viewing of the anterior chamber angle, turn the patient's head away from you (the surgeon) approximately 35° and turn the microscope toward you by approximately 35° (70° total). Position the gonioprism on the cornea to visualize the trabecular meshwork and ensure that a good view of the targeted implant site is available at the nasal implant location. To mitigate difficulty with patient movement or noncompliance, consider using a peri-bulbar or retro-bulbar block.

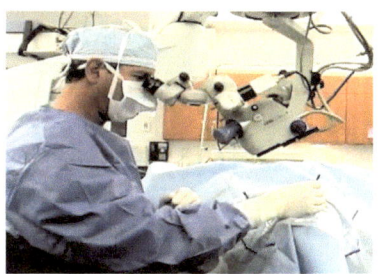

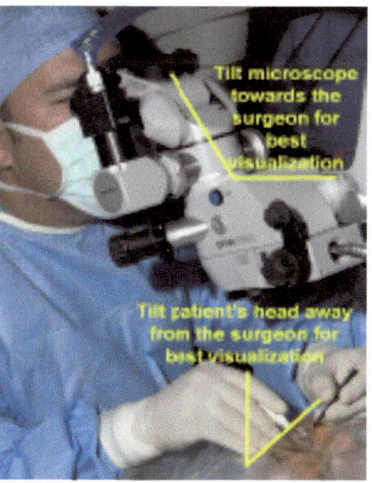

Step 2: Adjusting Microscope and Identifying Landmarks

Adjust the microscope setting to 10–12× and zoom and focus to locate the trabecular meshwork and identify the targeted stent implantation site. To visualize the targeted stent implantation location for the iStent Trabecular Micro-Bypass Stent and the iStent *inject*, focus on the landmarks shown in the image below and look anterior from the iris plane to find the scleral spur. The trabecular meshwork is located anterior to the scleral spur and is typically red/brown in color. Schlemm's canal is behind the trabecular meshwork.

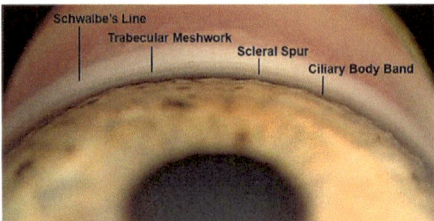 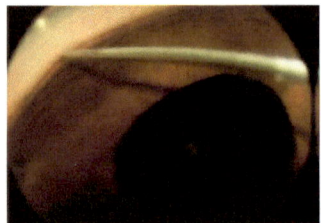

Step 3: Accessing Anterior Chamber

Deepen the anterior chamber with a cohesive viscoelastic as needed to maintain the chamber. When stent implantation is being performed with cataract surgery, enter the eye through the same corneal incision, otherwise create a 1.5 mm clear corneal incision for stent insertion. Hold the injector with your index finger comfortably on the micro-insertion sleeve retractor and within reach of the delivery button. Guide the micro-insertion tube across the anterior chamber just beyond the pupillary margin and then slide back the micro-insertion sleeve retractor (teal colored) to expose the micro-insertion tube and trocar. Replace the gonioprism, taking care to avoid contact with the lens or cornea.

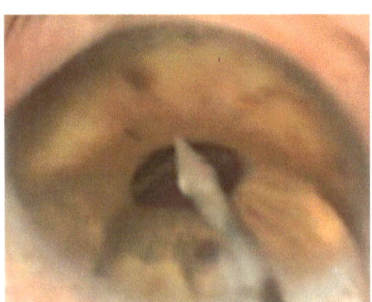 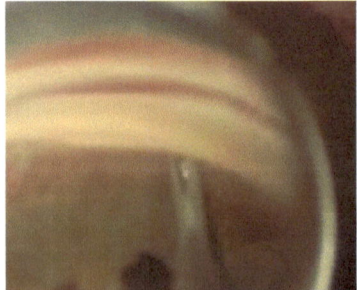

Step 4: Accessing Implantation Site

Locate the trabecular meshwork and select an implant location (shown below). Place the injector perpendicular to the trabecular meshwork and penetrate the tissue with the trocar.

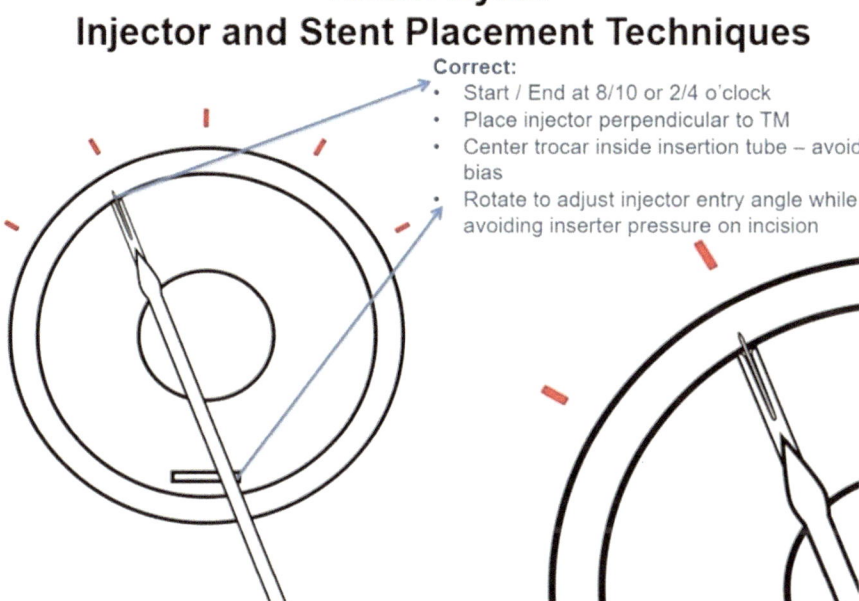

iStent *inject*
Injector and Stent Placement Techniques

Correct:
- Start / End at 8/10 or 2/4 o'clock
- Place injector perpendicular to TM
- Center trocar inside insertion tube – avoid bias
- Rotate to adjust injector entry angle while avoiding inserter pressure on incision

Step 5: Stent Implantation

Apply light pressure to the trabecular meshwork or dimple the tissue enough to see a "V" when pressing on the trabecular meshwork. Hold steady then deploy the stent by squeezing the stent delivery button with your index finger. A single audible click will indicate that the first stent has been delivered from the injector through the meshwork and into Schlemm's canal.

Before withdrawing the injector, look through the micro-insertion tube window during stent implantation to verify the stent is securely in place within the tissue. To withdraw the injector, hold the stent delivery button down and carefully withdraw the injector from the trabecular meshwork prior to releasing your finger from the stent delivery button. Upon release of the stent delivery button, a second audible click will indicate that the next stent is in position and ready to deliver.

While remaining in the eye, carefully move the injector at least 2 clock-hours away from the first implanted stent; approach the trabecular meshwork using the same technique. Squeeze the stent delivery button to deploy the second stent and remove the injector from the eye.

Confirm proper placement of the two implanted stents, ensuring that each stent flange is visible in the anterior chamber. Minimal blood reflux is a normal physiological response to stent placement, although this does not occur in all cases.

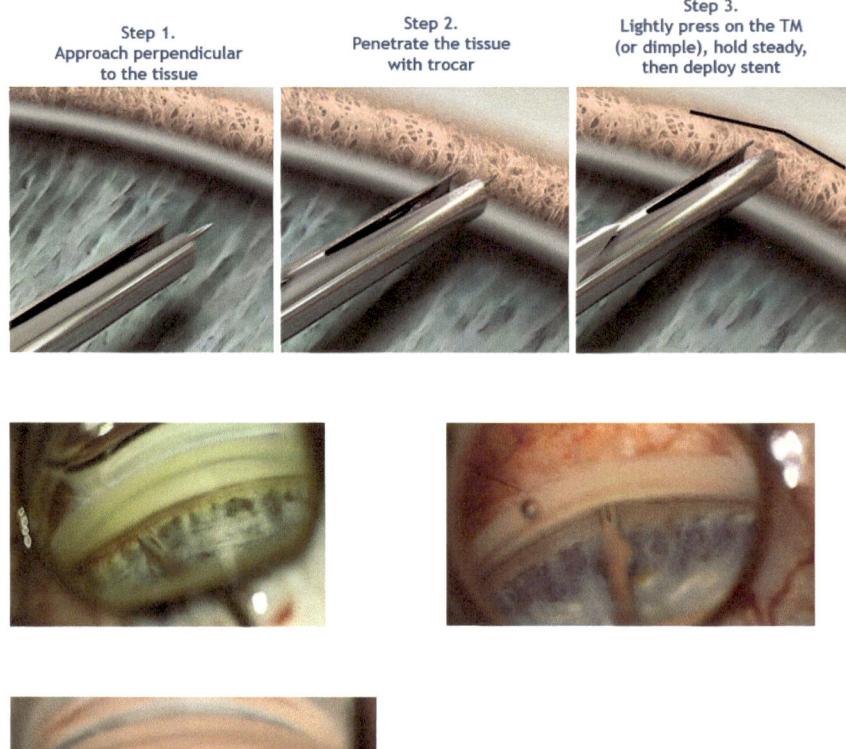

Step 1.
Approach perpendicular
to the tissue

Step 2.
Penetrate the tissue
with trocar

Step 3.
Lightly press on the TM
(or dimple), hold steady,
then deploy stent

Step 6: Viscoelastic Removal

Using the corneal incision, irrigate and aspirate the anterior chamber with balanced salt solution (BSS) to remove all viscoelastic, pressing down on the posterior edge of the incision to facilitate complete removal of viscoelastic. Repeat as needed until all viscoelastic has been removed. Inflate the anterior chamber with saline solution to achieve physiologic pressure. Ensure that the corneal incision is sealed.

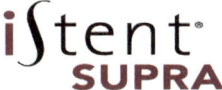

Step 1: Patient Positioning and Setup

To obtain proper viewing of the anterior chamber angle, turn the patient's head away from you (the surgeon) approximately 35° and turn the microscope toward you by approximately 35° (70° total). Position the gonioprism on the cornea to visualize the anterior chamber angle and ensure that a good view is available at the implant location. To mitigate difficulty with patient movement or noncompliance, consider using a peri-bulbar or retro-bulbar block.

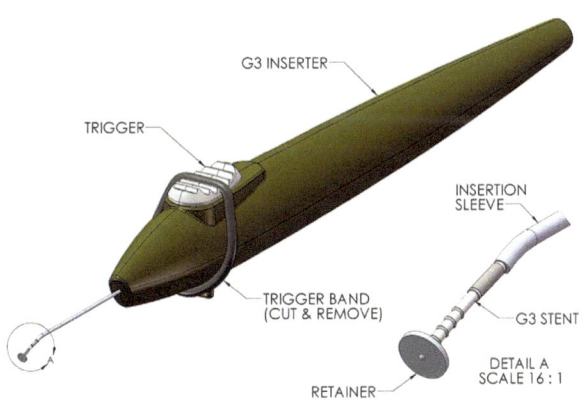

© The Author(s) 2021

C. C. A. Sng, K. Barton (eds.), *Minimally Invasive Glaucoma Surgery*,

https://doi.org/10.1007/978-981-15-5632-6

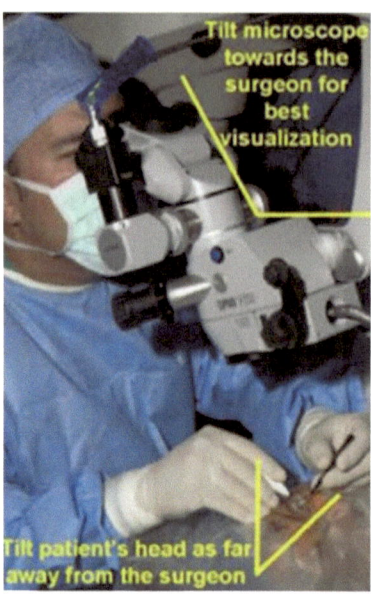

Step 2: Adjusting Microscope and Identifying Landmarks

Adjust the microscope setting to 10–12× and zoom and focus to the targeted stent implantation site. To visualize the targeted stent implantation site for the iStent SUPRA, focus on the landmarks shown in the image below and look anterior from the iris plane to find the scleral spur. The suprachoroidal space is located inferior to the scleral spur.

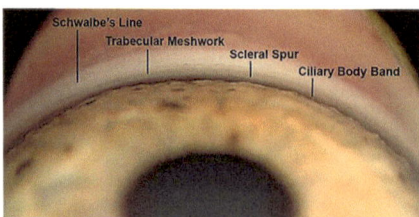

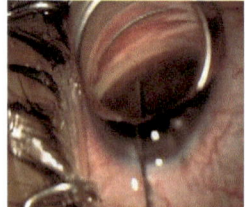

Step 3: Accessing Anterior Chamber

Deepen the anterior chamber with a cohesive viscoelastic as needed to maintain the chamber and coat the tip of the inserter with a small drop of viscoelastic. When stent implantation is being performed with cataract surgery, enter the eye through the same corneal incision, otherwise create a 1.5 mm clear corneal incision for stent insertion. Enter the anterior chamber and advance across the pupillary margin before replacing the gonioprism, taking care to avoid contact with the lens or cornea.

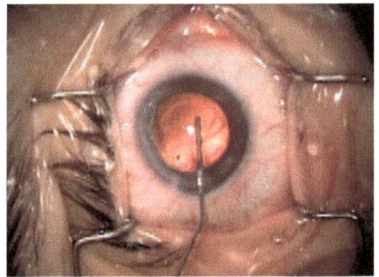
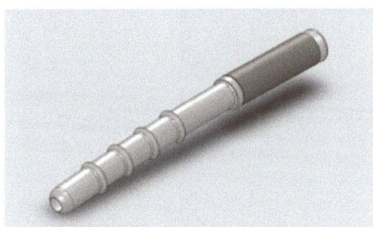

Step 4: Accessing Implantation Site

Create a narrow passage into the suprachoroidal space by gently separating the iris processes away from the scleral spur with the tip of the insertion trocar until the anterior and posterior portions of the sclera spur are fully visible on a very limited area (create an approximately 0.5 mm to a maximum of 1 mm width opening). If needed, a spatula may be used for this step. Limited bleeding may occur if the spatula contacts capillary vasculature structure; if blood obscures the view of the implantation site, use viscoelastic to clear the view.

Advance the iStent SUPRA until the anterior surface of the stent is tangent to the posterior margin of the scleral spur. With your finger firmly on the inserter trigger in the forward position, carefully advance the trocar/stent into the suprachoroidal space until the titanium sleeve just passes the scleral spur and enters the suprachoroidal space. Ensure that approximately half (or 0.4–0.7 mm) of the sleeve portion remains in the anterior chamber.

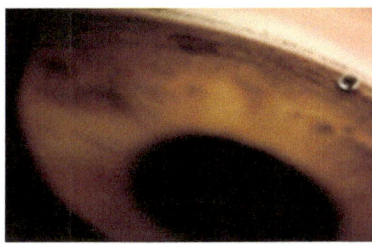
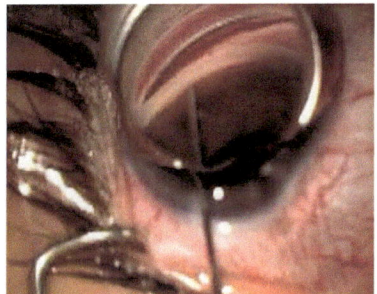

Step 5: Stent Implantation

Once the stent is in the correct position at the proper depth, carefully slide the trigger button backward until the stent is released and withdraw the inserter from eye. Use the operating microscope and gonioprism to confirm that the stent is in the proper position where the proximal end rests in the anterior chamber with an unobstructed inlet.

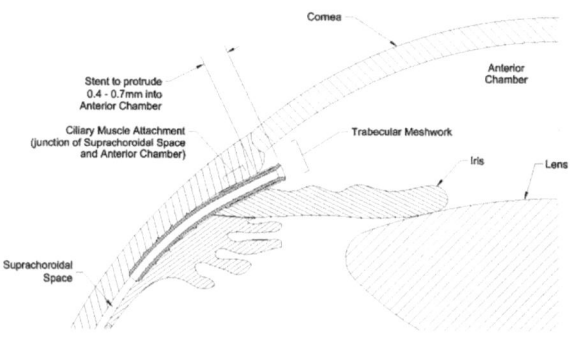

Step 6: Viscoelastic Removal

Using the corneal incision, irrigate and aspirate the anterior chamber with balanced salt solution (BSS) to remove all viscoelastic, pressing down on the posterior edge of the incision to facilitate complete removal of viscoelastic. Repeat as needed until all viscoelastic has been removed. Inflate the anterior chamber with saline solution to achieve physiologic pressure. Ensure that the corneal incision is sealed.

Appendix D: Trabectome

Narrative Instructions by NeoMedix Corporation

Equipment

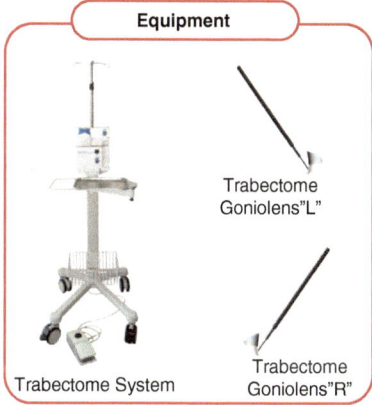

Trabectome System

Trabectome Goniolens"L"

Trabectome Goniolens"R"

Procesure Pack

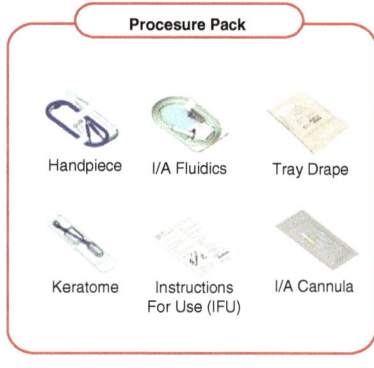

Handpiece

I/A Fluidics

Tray Drape

Keratome

Instructions For Use (IFU)

I/A Cannula

Step 1: Clear Corneal Incision

Create a 1.8-mm clear corneal incision with slit knife. Flare the incision on the inside to extend the reach toward the left and the right and prevent corneal folds.

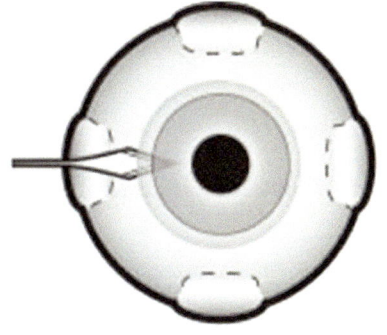

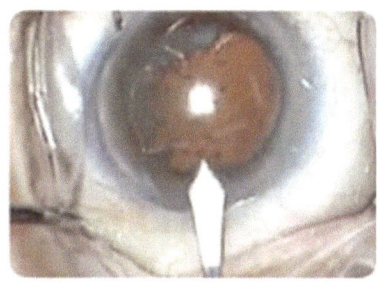

© The Author(s) 2021
C. C. A. Sng, K. Barton (eds.), *Minimally Invasive Glaucoma Surgery*,
https://doi.org/10.1007/978-981-15-5632-6

It is recommended that Trabectome surgery is performed prior to cataract surgery for the best corneal clarity. However, if cataract surgery is performed before Trabectome surgery, it is advisable to suture the corneal incision, so as to decrease the size of the incision and reduce leak during Trabectome surgery.

Step 2: Lower Anterior Chamber Intraocular Pressure to Visualize Schlemm's Canal

Open the corneal incision to allow aqueous humor to leave the anterior chamber, lowering intraocular pressure. Blood reflux into Schlemm's Canal will then promote visualization of the trabecular meshwork. The anterior chamber is reformed by injecting balanced salt solution.

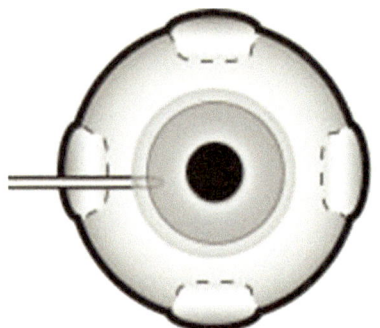 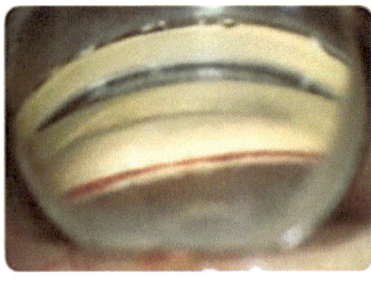

Step 3: Microscope Tilt and Head

The microscope is tilted toward the surgeon by approximately 40° and the microscope oculars are repositioned. Sitting temporally, the patient's head is rotated away by approximately 30°. The best view of the trabecular meshwork is achieved when the angle of the microscope and the patient's eye equals 70°.

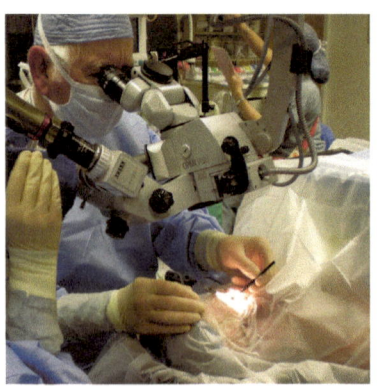 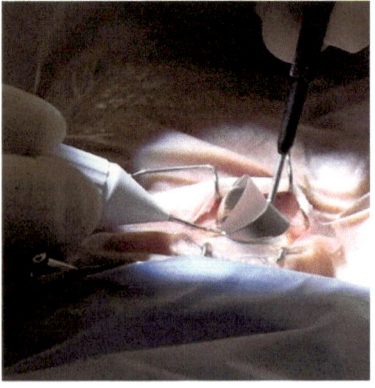

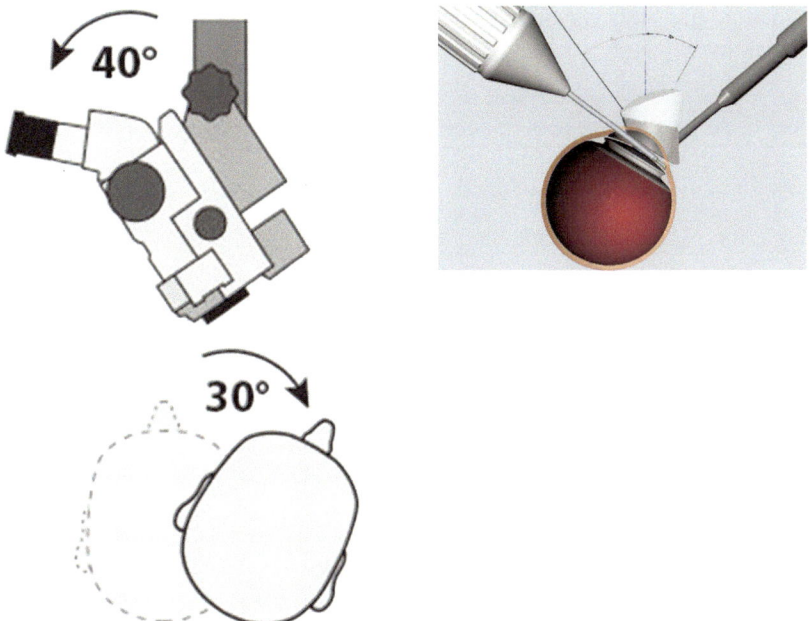

Step 4: Goniolens Placement

Place the goniolens on the cornea and identify the trabecular meshwork (enhanced by Step 2). Ensure that the correct goniolens is used (handle on the left for right-handed surgeons and handle on the right for left-handed surgeons). Remove the Goniolens and inset the tip with irrigation on. Advance the tip three-quarters of the way across the anterior chamber toward the trabecular meshwork, then replace the Goniolens and continue advancing tip, contacting trabecular meshwork. Float the goniolens on the cornea and do not compress to avoid striae. Do not use viscoelastic to pressurize the eye.

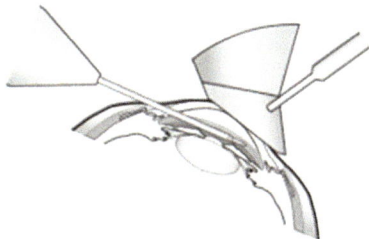

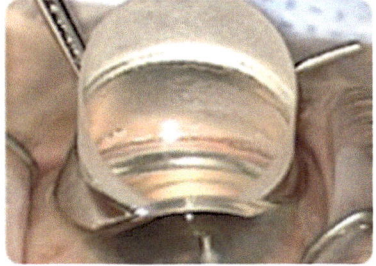

Favorable and less favorable Trabectome handpiece grip techniques are shown below:

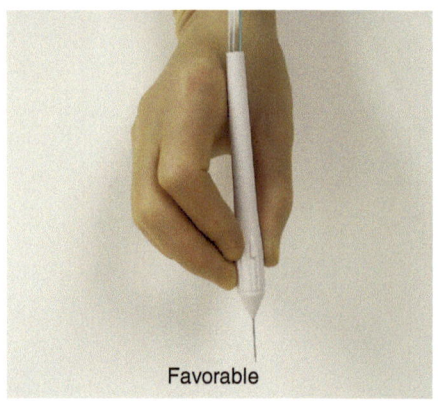

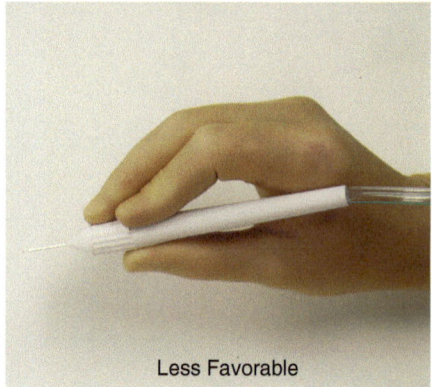

| Favorable | Less Favorable |

Step 5: Removal of Trabecular Meshwork

Gently insert the tip into Schlemm's Canal highlighted with blood congestion. Depress the foot pedal to activate aspiration and electrosurgical power. Advance the Trabectome tip clockwise within Schlemm's Canal to remove trabecular meshwork. Bring the Trabectome tip in the center of the anterior chamber and rotate 180°, then repeat in a counterclockwise direction to remove the trabecular meshwork. Ablate as much as you can safely ablate (up to 180° using one incision).

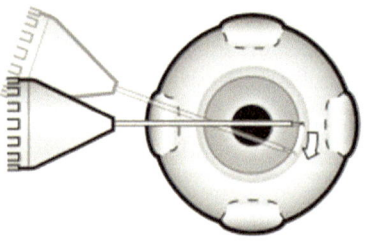

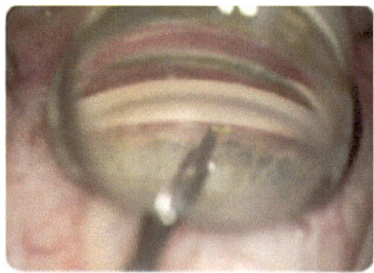

When entering the TM:
1. Visual contact with trabecular meshwork
2. Minimal pressure and gentle compression of trabecular meshwork
3. Enter tip through wrinkle in trabecular meshwork arcing into Schlemm's Canal
4. Slowly advance tip in Schlemm's Canal to take out the middle third of the width of the trabecular meshwork

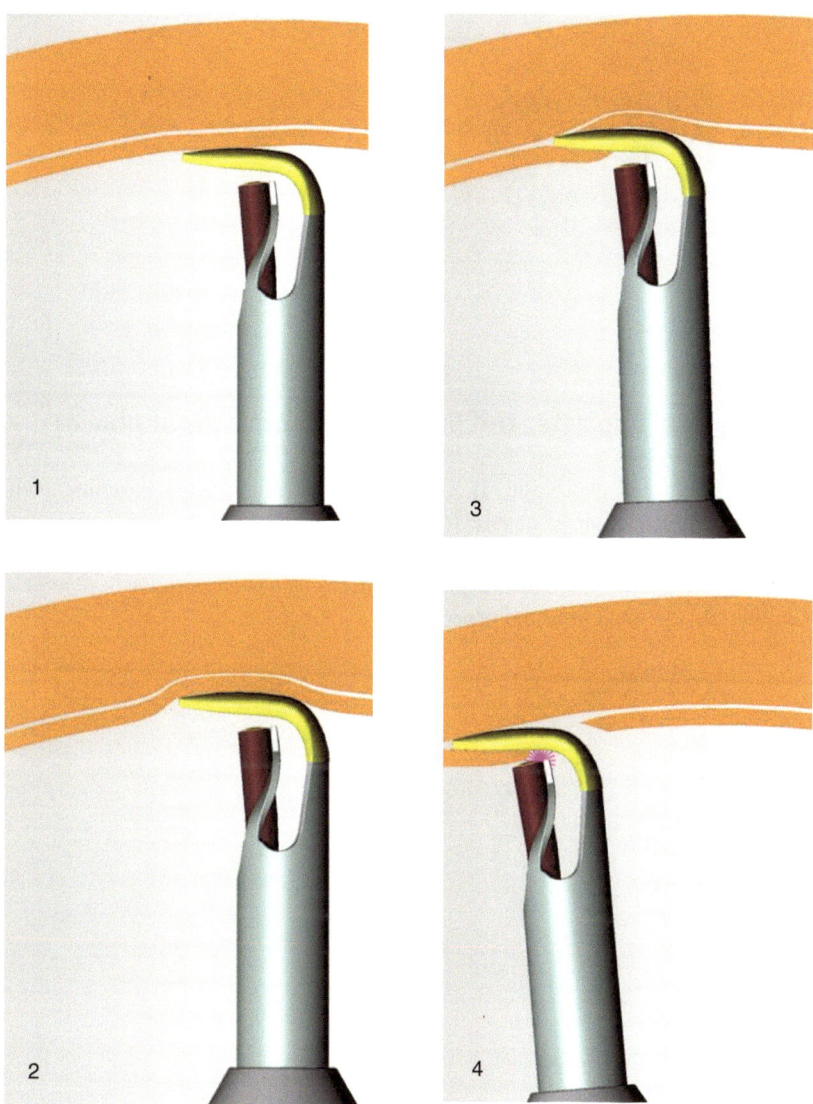

When removing the trabecular meshwork, ablate along the arc, pointing the tip of the footplate forward and power during rotation along the arc, with the footplate within Schlemm's Canal acting as a guide. Ensure that there is continual handpiece withdrawal toward the surgeon to minimize friction on the posterior wall of Schlemm's Canal while advancing along the arc, which would damage the collector channels.

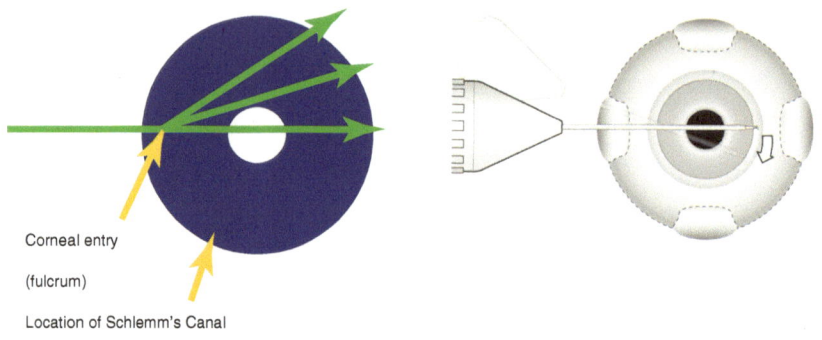

Corneal entry

(fulcrum)

Location of Schlemm's Canal

Step 6: Irrigate, Aspirate, and Suture (With or Without Phaco)

Perform irrigation and aspiration. If Trabectome surgery is NOT combined with Phaco, suture the incision to ensure leak-tight closure. If Trabectome surgery is combined with Phaco, enlarge the incision and proceed with Phaco, intraocular lens insertion then suture to ensure leak-tight closure. Reduce postoperative hyphema by pressurizing the eye well after the procedure.

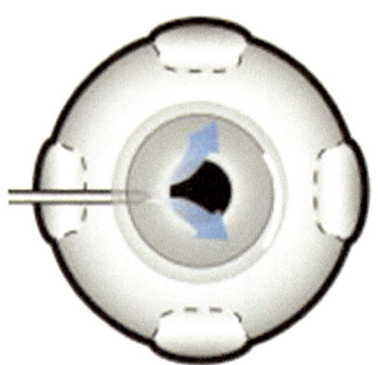
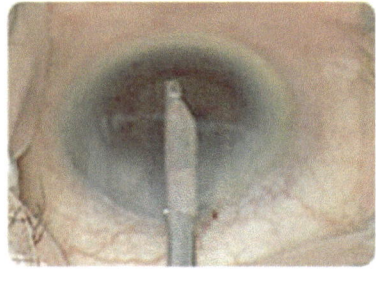

Appendix E: Hydrus Microstent Procedure Steps

Narrative Instructions By Ivantis, Inc.

Step 1

After completion of cataract surgery, or as stand-alone approach, adjust the patient's head and surgical microscope to the proper position to assure an adequate view of the angle of the eye using a gonioscopic prism lens.

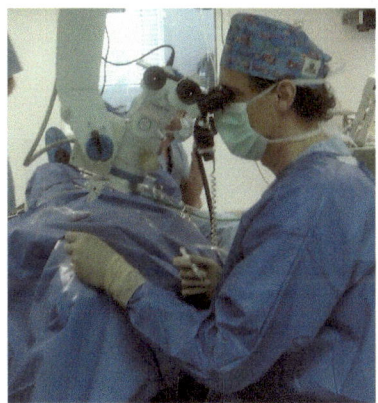

Step 2

Fill the anterior chamber with a cohesive OVD.

© The Author(s) 2021
C. C. A. Sng, K. Barton (eds.), *Minimally Invasive Glaucoma Surgery*,
https://doi.org/10.1007/978-981-15-5632-6

Step 3

Using gonioscopy, confirm that the angle is open and the angle structures are suitable for microstent implantation.

Step 4

The surgeon should be able to clearly identify the scleral spur and the trabecular meshwork (TM).

Step 5

Use an existing (or create a new) clear cornea incision (minimum of 2 mm) to insert the Hydrus delivery cannula.

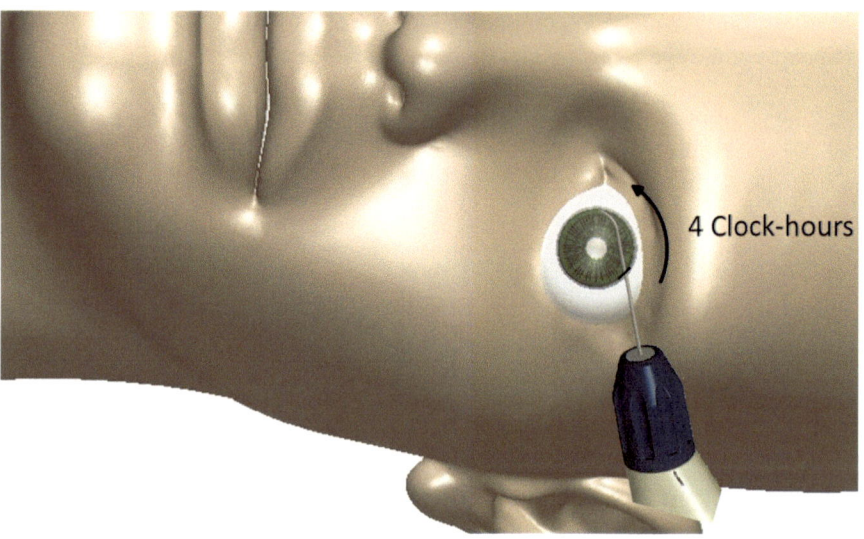

Step 6

Advance the Hydrus delivery cannula under gonioscopic guidance and approach the TM with the cannula tip at a slight upward angle.

Target the pigmented TM for cannula tip insertion

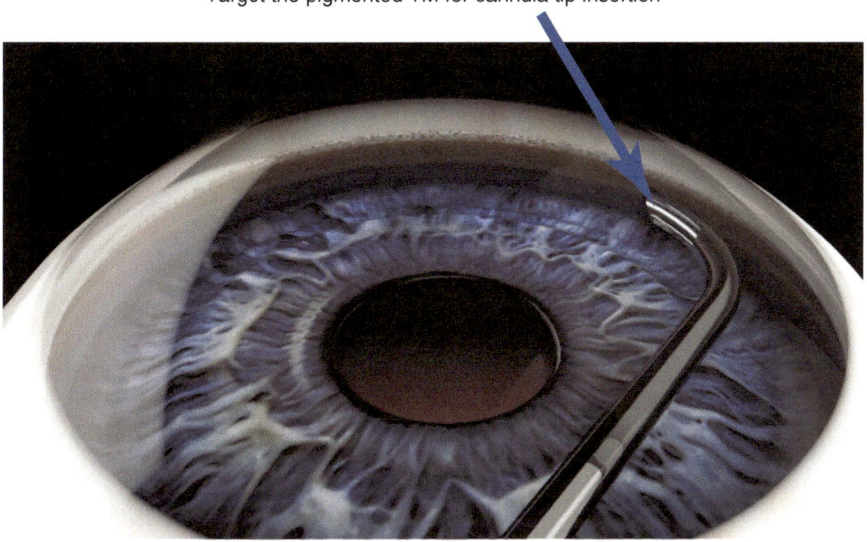

Step 7

Penetrate the TM so that the beveled portion of the cannula tip is completely through the TM and position the back of the cannula tip against the posterior wall of Schlemm's canal (Fig. 3). Use the tracking wheel on the delivery system to slowly advance and implant the Hydrus Microstent, while keeping the cannula tip firmly in place. As the Hydrus implant advances, relax any upward or posterior pressure, while continuing to keep the cannula tip in place. An interlock mechanism will release from the microstent inlet when the tracking wheel is fully advanced. The interlock mechanism leaves the inlet in the anterior chamber, while the microstent scaffold resides in Schlemm's canal, dilating the canal in a 90° span and providing enhanced aqueous access to multiple major collector channels.

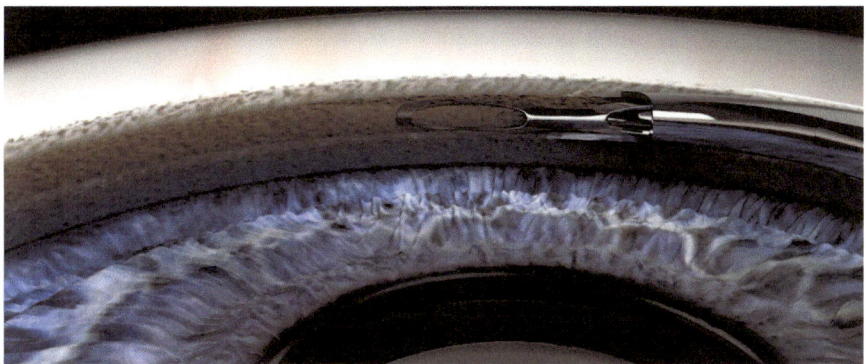

Step 8

Visual confirmation of the microstent through the TM results in confidence of device placement.

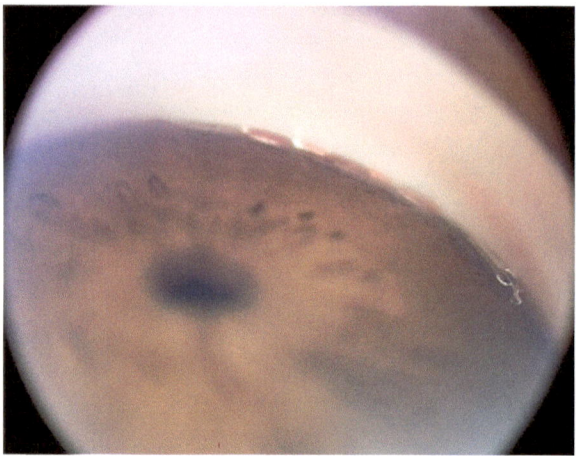

The microstent position can be adjusted if necessary with surgical micrograspers. The microstent can be recaptured and removed using the delivery system and it's tracking wheel in a reverse direction. If recapture is necessary, place the cannula tip behind the microstent inlet with the interlock mechanism in front of the inlet. Using the tracking wheel in reverse direction will result in the interlock mechanism capturing the microstent inlet and retrieving the implant into the delivery cannula.

Step 9

Following successful microstent implantation, remove OVD and close eye per standard procedure.

Appendix F: XEN Gel Implant

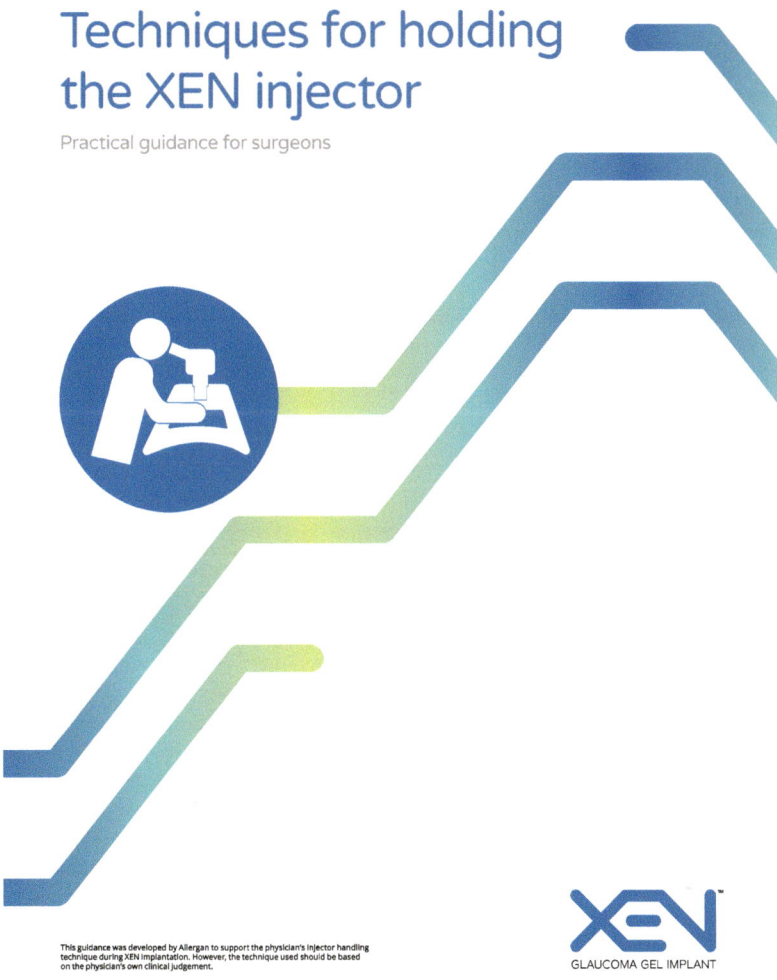

Techniques for holding the XEN injector

Practical guidance for surgeons

XEN™
GLAUCOMA GEL IMPLANT

© The Author(s) 2021
C. C. A. Sng, K. Barton (eds.), *Minimally Invasive Glaucoma Surgery*,
https://doi.org/10.1007/978-981-15-5632-6

How to hold the XEN injector and avoid common errors

This guidance has been developed by Allergan to help
you refine your technique and avoid common errors

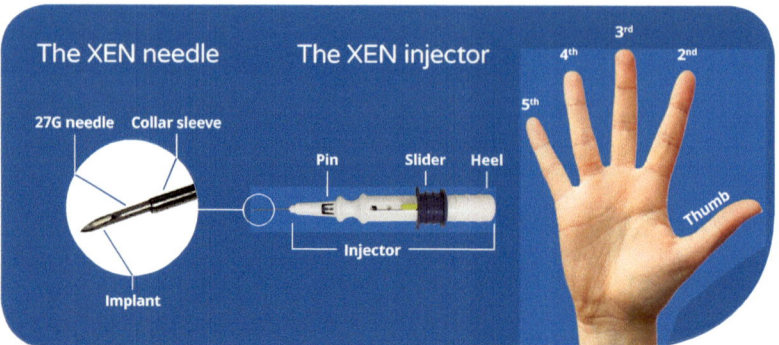

We recommend using one of these three implantation techniques:

1 Superior seating position

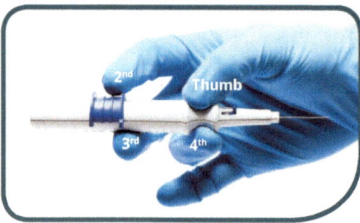

Hold the injector between the
thumb and 4ᵗʰ finger

Use the **3ʳᵈ finger** to support
the underside of the injector

Use the **2ⁿᵈ finger** to deploy the slider

The injector needle should point towards the wrist

Keep the injector in a horizontal position

When entering the eye, the **2ⁿᵈ finger** should rest
in front of the slider to avoid accidental deployment

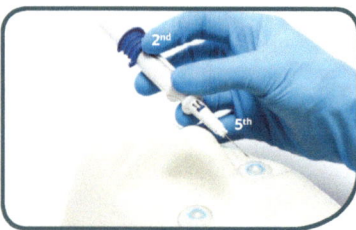

The **5ᵗʰ finger** can be positioned on
the patient's cheek for added stability

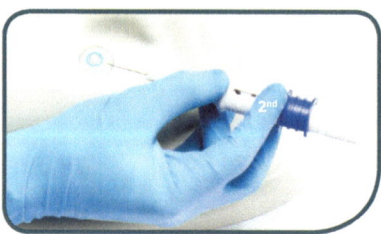

The wrist should be kept as straight as possible

Move the **2ⁿᵈ finger** onto the slider once the needle
bevel is visible in the subconjunctival space

2 Temporal seating position – overhand

Hold the injector between the **2nd and 3rd fingers**
The injector needle should point away from the wrist

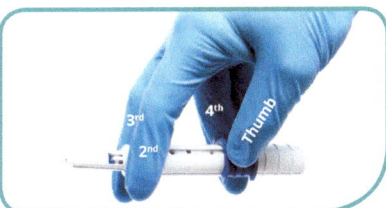 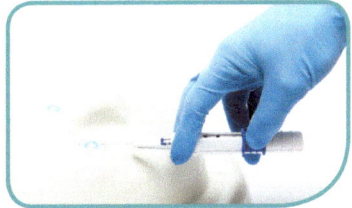

Keep the injector in a horizontal position
Use the **4th finger** to support the injector
Use the **thumb** to deploy the slider

Keeping the wrist as straight as possible will aid movement of the **thumb** (slider)

It may be necessary to elevate the arm at the elbow to relax the wrist

3 Temporal seating position – underhand

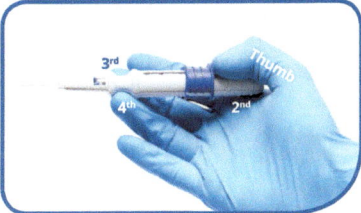

Rest the injector between the **3rd and 4th fingers**

Position the heel of the injector between the **2nd finger and thumb**

Use the **thumb** to grip the heel of the injector and to deploy the slider when required

The injector needle should point away from the wrist

Keep the injector in a horizontal position

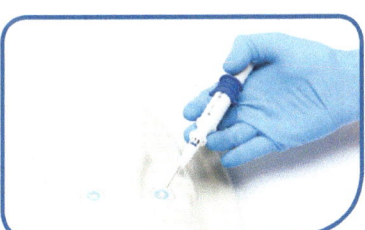 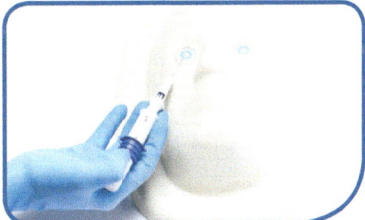

Turning the palm of the hand upwards will improve access to the superonasal quadrant

The **thumb** should be able to comfortably reach the end of the slider track without becoming over strained or destabilising the injector

Common errors you should try and avoid when implanting XEN

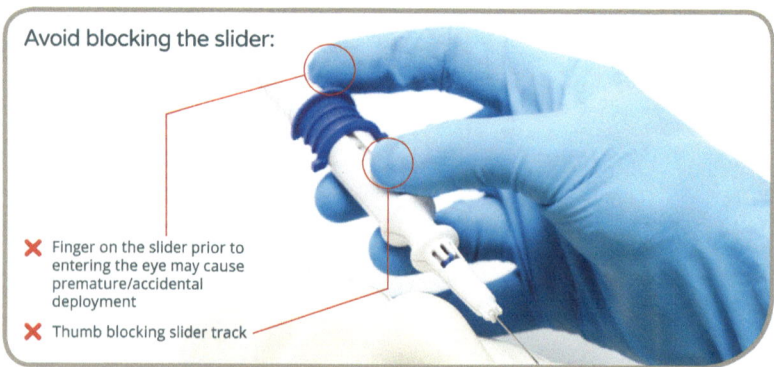

Avoid blocking the slider:

✗ Finger on the slider prior to entering the eye may cause premature/accidental deployment

✗ Thumb blocking slider track

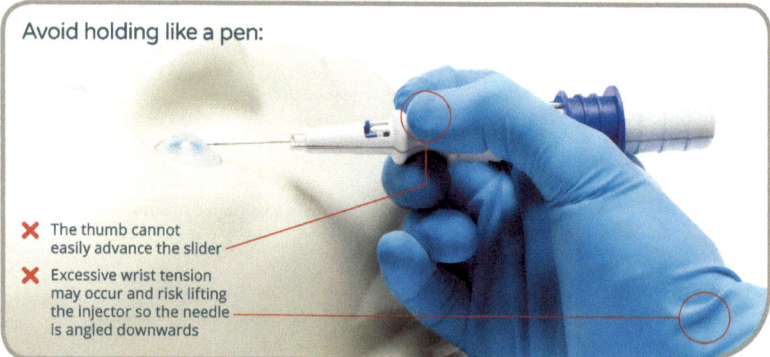

Avoid holding like a pen:

✗ The thumb cannot easily advance the slider

✗ Excessive wrist tension may occur and risk lifting the injector so the needle is angled downwards

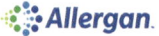

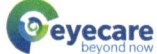

Mastering XEN

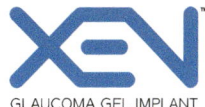

Mastering XEN[1]

1

Plan XEN location before making incisions

- Plan the main and side port
- Mark the target zone
- Check for injector clearance
- Rotate the speculum
- Practise with the goniolens

2

Advance needle through sclera

- Stop and confirm needle tip exit at 3 +/- 0.5 mm
- Pull all the way back and re-enter at a higher or lower angle, if needed

3

Continue to advance the needle

- Confirm that full bevel is visible
- Rotate the bevel 90° towards 12 o'clock
- Use high magnification view

4

Deliver XEN through gentle actuation of slider

- Maintain slight forward pressure on injector
- As the needle withdraws into the sleeve, neutralise side pressure or any needle bending

5

Confirm XEN position in subconjunctival space and anterior chamber

- Use high magnification
- If long in anterior chamber (>2 mm) or short in subconjunctival space (<2 mm), adjust from outside, or remove from anterior chamber side and place new implant

Confirm significant bleb with priming

- Remove viscoelastic starting at XEN
- Straighten curled implant with dull instrument
- If not connected in anterior chamber, gently push XEN back into the anterior chamber

6

Monitoring patients

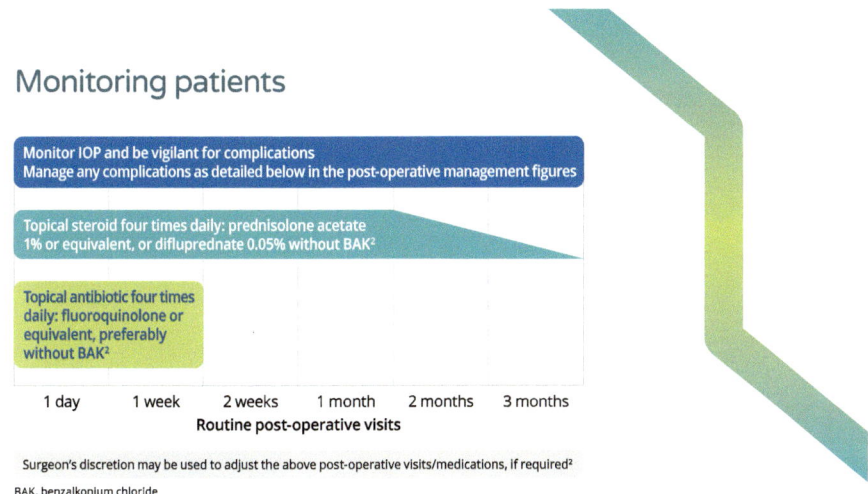

Monitor IOP and be vigilant for complications
Manage any complications as detailed below in the post-operative management figures

Topical steroid four times daily: prednisolone acetate
1% or equivalent, or difluprednate 0.05% without BAK[2]

Topical antibiotic four times daily: fluoroquinolone or equivalent, preferably without BAK[2]

| 1 day | 1 week | 2 weeks | 1 month | 2 months | 3 months |

Routine post-operative visits

Surgeon's discretion may be used to adjust the above post-operative visits/medications, if required[2]

BAK, benzalkonium chloride

Post-operative management: day one to week one[3]

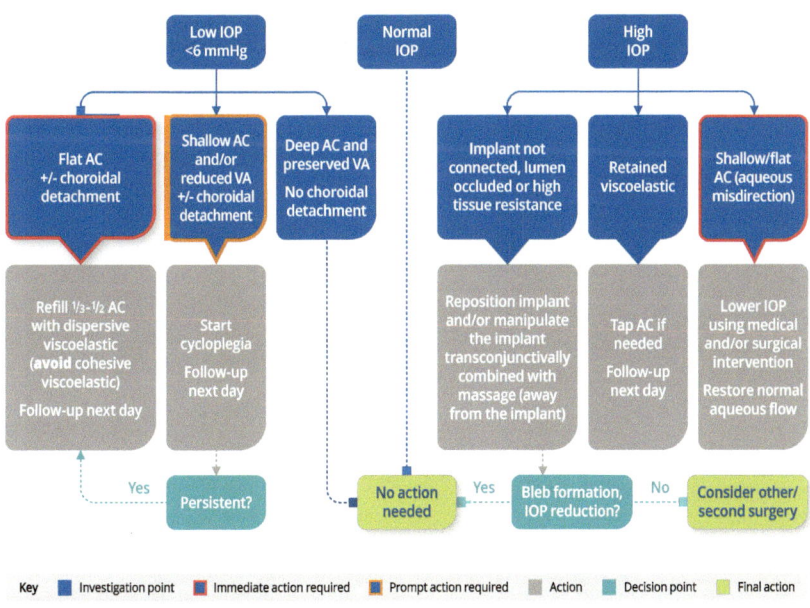

Key: Investigation point | Immediate action required | Prompt action required | Action | Decision point | Final action

AC, anterior chamber; IOP, intraocular pressure; VA, visual acuity

This guidance was created via consensus from an expert meeting funded by Allergan. It has been developed for the sole purpose of providing scientific information and is designed to support the physician's decision making process, however, the final decision should be based on their own clinical judgement.

Post-operative management:
after one week, assuming implant connection is confirmed[3]

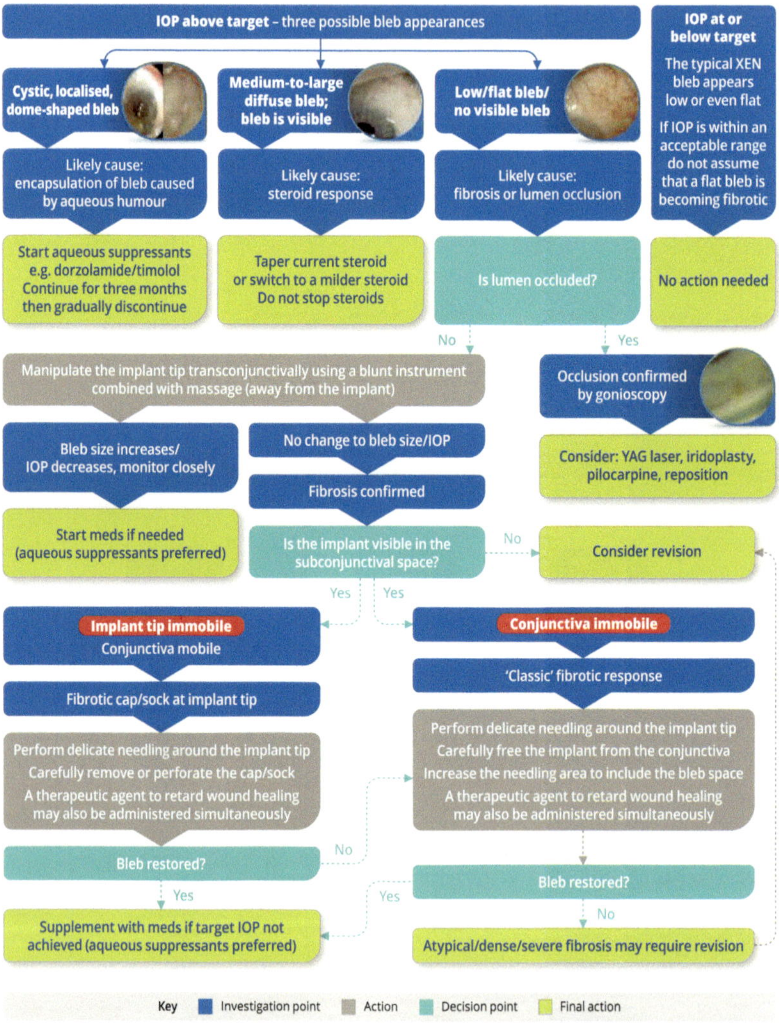

IOP above target – three possible bleb appearances

IOP at or below target

The typical XEN bleb appears low or even flat

Cystic, localised, dome-shaped bleb

Medium-to-large diffuse bleb; bleb is visible

Low/flat bleb/ no visible bleb

If IOP is within an acceptable range do not assume that a flat bleb is becoming fibrotic

Likely cause: encapsulation of bleb caused by aqueous humour

Likely cause: steroid response

Likely cause: fibrosis or lumen occlusion

Start aqueous suppressants e.g. dorzolamide/timolol Continue for three months then gradually discontinue

Taper current steroid or switch to a milder steroid Do not stop steroids

Is lumen occluded?

No action needed

No   Yes

Manipulate the implant tip transconjunctivally using a blunt instrument combined with massage (away from the implant)

Occlusion confirmed by gonioscopy

Bleb size increases/ IOP decreases, monitor closely

No change to bleb size/IOP

Consider: YAG laser, iridoplasty, pilocarpine, reposition

Fibrosis confirmed

Start meds if needed (aqueous suppressants preferred)

Is the implant visible in the subconjunctival space?

No

Consider revision

Yes   Yes

Implant tip immobile
Conjunctiva mobile

Conjunctiva immobile

'Classic' fibrotic response

Fibrotic cap/sock at implant tip

Perform delicate needling around the implant tip
Carefully remove or perforate the cap/sock
A therapeutic agent to retard wound healing may also be administered simultaneously

Perform delicate needling around the implant tip
Carefully free the implant from the conjunctiva
Increase the needling area to include the bleb space
A therapeutic agent to retard wound healing may also be administered simultaneously

Bleb restored?

No

Yes

Bleb restored?

Yes

Supplement with meds if target IOP not achieved (aqueous suppressants preferred)

No

Atypical/dense/severe fibrosis may require revision

Key   ■ Investigation point   ■ Action   ■ Decision point   ■ Final action

This guidance was created via consensus from an expert meeting funded by Allergan. It has been developed for the sole purpose of providing scientific information and is designed to support the physician's decision making process, however, the final decision should be based on their own clinical judgement.

1. Allergan Data on file INT/0511/2017 July 2017. Marlow, UK.
2. Allergan Data on file INT/0175/2015 January 2016. Marlow, UK.
3. Allergan Data on file INT/0126/2017 March 2017. Marlow, UK.

The XEN gel implant is intended to reduce intraocular pressure in patients with primary open angle glaucoma where previous medical treatments have failed. XEN is a medical device class III CE 0086. Always refer to the full instructions before use.

Adverse events should be reported to your local regulatory office and your Allergan office.

Date of preparation: July 2017 INT/0189/2017a(1)

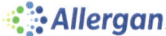

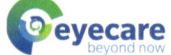

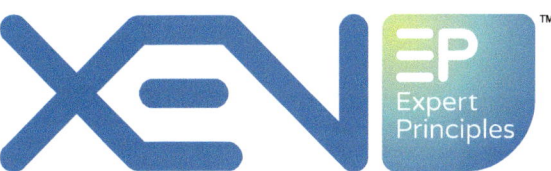

Introducing
XEN Expert Principles (EP)

**Developed in collaboration with leading surgeons
to highlight the most important elements
of XEN implantation**

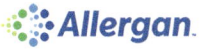

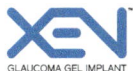

GLAUCOMA GEL IMPLANT

This guidance was created via consensus from XEN experts funded by Allergan. It has been developed for the sole purpose of
providing additional practical XEN implantation techniques and is designed to support the physician's decision making process,
however, the final decision and technique used should be based on their own clinical judgement.

What is XEN-EP?

The guiding principles of XEN-EP apply at every stage of implantation. These are:

Control inflammation

The four stages of XEN-EP | **Stage objectives**

Intra-operative

Preparation — Healthy conjunctiva and hydroexpansion

- Control ocular surface and lid margin inflammation and hyperaemia by using pre-operative steroids if necessary
- Avoid conjunctival trauma when preparing the patient
- Select a form of anaesthesia that avoids any sensation of pain or discomfort for the patient

Placement — Perfectly positioned implant

- Avoid causing trauma to the iris and angle structures with the XEN injector

Priming — Flowing and free

- Remove all blood from the anterior chamber

Post-operative

Post-op — 'START LOW STAY LOW'

- Topical steroid medications for one month and taper
- Topical antibiotics for one week

Lower conjunctival outflow resistance

Minimise bleeding

Hydroexpand the Tenon layer by injecting 0.1 ml fluid approximately 5-8 mm posterior to the limbus

'Balloon' the bleb area with fluid, then migrate the fluid posteriorly

Avoid fluid pooling at the limbus

Take care to avoid blood vessels when introducing the needle

Use vasoconstrictors if the eye appears hyperaemic

Control bleeding via tamponade if it occurs

Use a small needle (30 G/insulin) for hydroexpansion

Position the implant in a healthy area of conjunctiva as close to 12 o'clock as possible

Create a '1-2-3' connection to permit outflow as posteriorly as possible:
1 mm anterior chamber
2 mm scleral channel
3 mm subconjunctival space

Position the injector needle entry anterior to Schlemm's canal

Carefully control the injector forces during implant deployment to avoid 'flicks' during needle retraction

Thoroughly remove all viscoelastic

Hydrate the incisions, pressurise the eye using balanced salt solution (sufficient to deepen the anterior chamber) and observe bleb formation

Verify the implant is straight and the tip is mobile

Leave the anterior chamber formed and stable

Carefully liberate immobile implants intra-operatively

Target day one IOP of 3-10 mmHg (optimal baseline IOP)

Measure the IOP at one week, assess the difference in IOP from day one (week one delta)

Based on the week one delta, consider supplementary measures to enhance outflow under the following conditions:
- IOP ≥14 mmHg and week one delta ≥6 mmHg
- IOP ≥16 mmHg
- IOP ≥ target IOP

Apply the principles described in the post-operative management guidance

Target needling at the most likely areas of outflow obstruction

Take care when needling not to cause bleeding or excessive tissue trauma

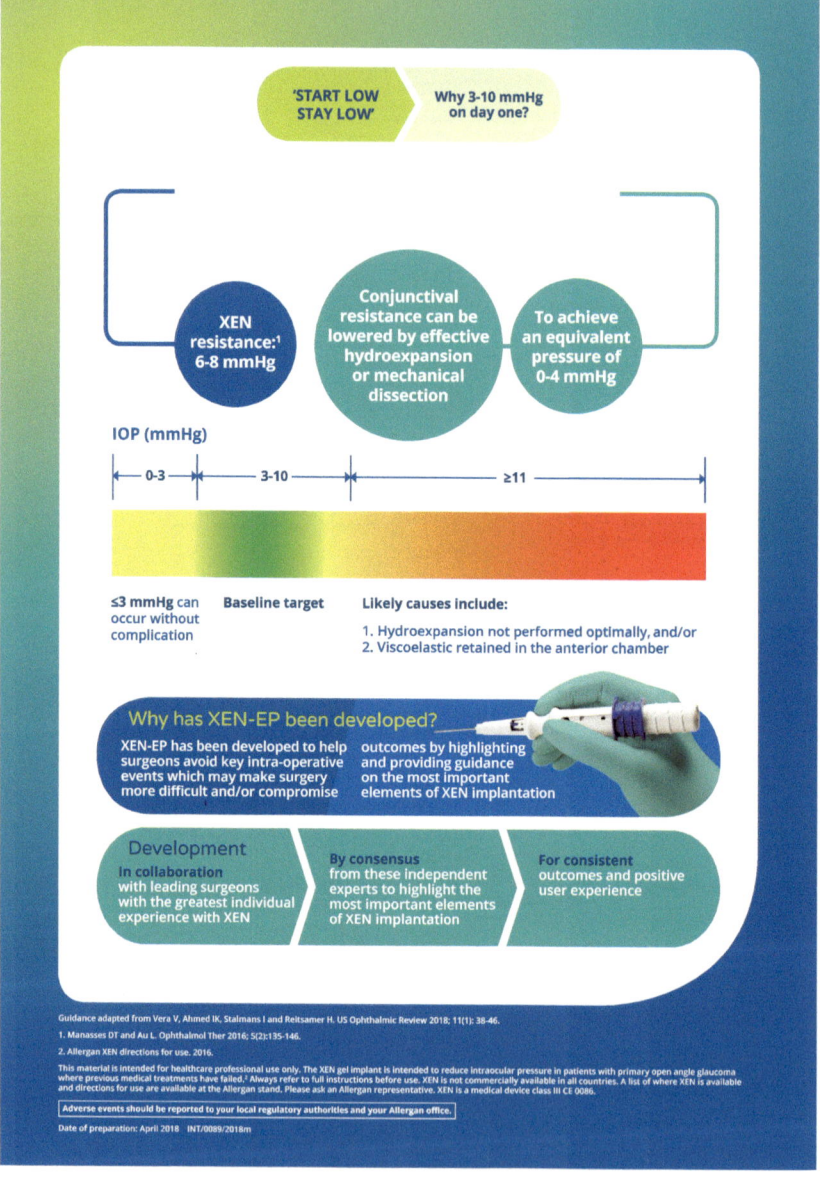

'START LOW STAY LOW' — Why 3-10 mmHg on day one?

XEN resistance:[1] 6-8 mmHg

Conjunctival resistance can be lowered by effective hydroexpansion or mechanical dissection

To achieve an equivalent pressure of 0-4 mmHg

IOP (mmHg)

0-3 — 3-10 — ≥11

≤3 mmHg can occur without complication

Baseline target

Likely causes include:

1. Hydroexpansion not performed optimally, and/or
2. Viscoelastic retained in the anterior chamber

Why has XEN-EP been developed?

XEN-EP has been developed to help surgeons avoid key intra-operative events which may make surgery more difficult and/or compromise outcomes by highlighting and providing guidance on the most important elements of XEN implantation

Development

In collaboration with leading surgeons with the greatest individual experience with XEN

By consensus from these independent experts to highlight the most important elements of XEN implantation

For consistent outcomes and positive user experience

Guidance adapted from Vera V, Ahmed IK, Stalmans I and Reitsamer H. US Ophthalmic Review 2018; 11(1): 38-46.

1. Manasses DT and Au L. Ophthalmol Ther 2016; 5(2):135-146.

2. Allergan XEN directions for use. 2016.

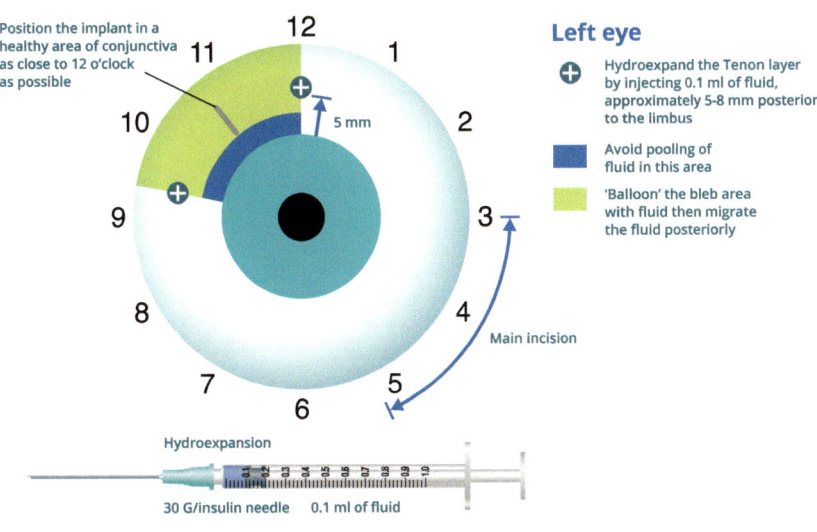

Position the implant in a healthy area of conjunctiva as close to 12 o'clock as possible

5 mm

Main incision

Hydroexpansion

30 G/insulin needle   0.1 ml of fluid

Left eye

⊕ Hydroexpand the Tenon layer by injecting 0.1 ml of fluid, approximately 5-8 mm posterior to the limbus

Avoid pooling of fluid in this area

'Balloon' the bleb area with fluid then migrate the fluid posteriorly

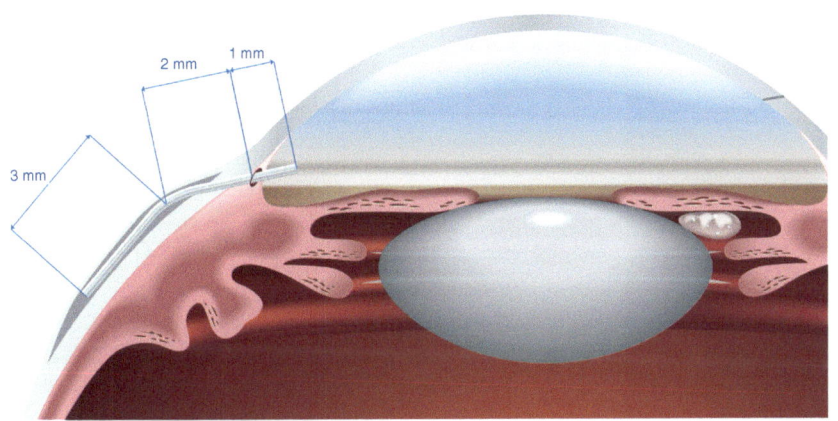

2 mm   1 mm

3 mm

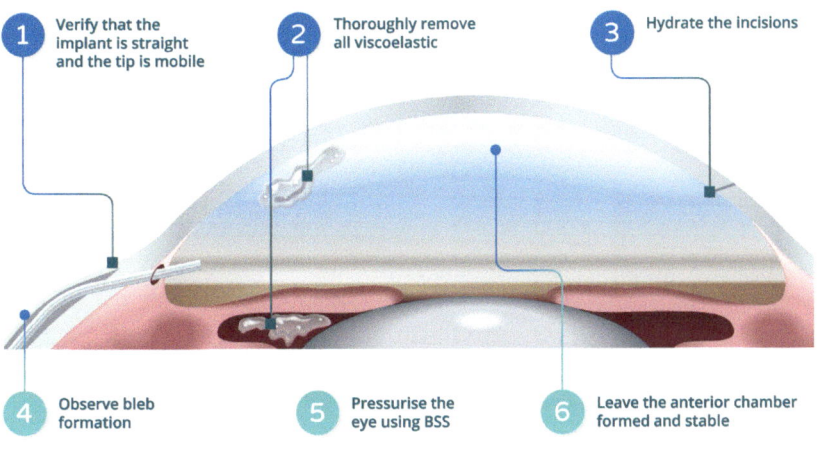

1 Verify that the implant is straight and the tip is mobile

2 Thoroughly remove all viscoelastic

3 Hydrate the incisions

4 Observe bleb formation

5 Pressurise the eye using BSS

6 Leave the anterior chamber formed and stable

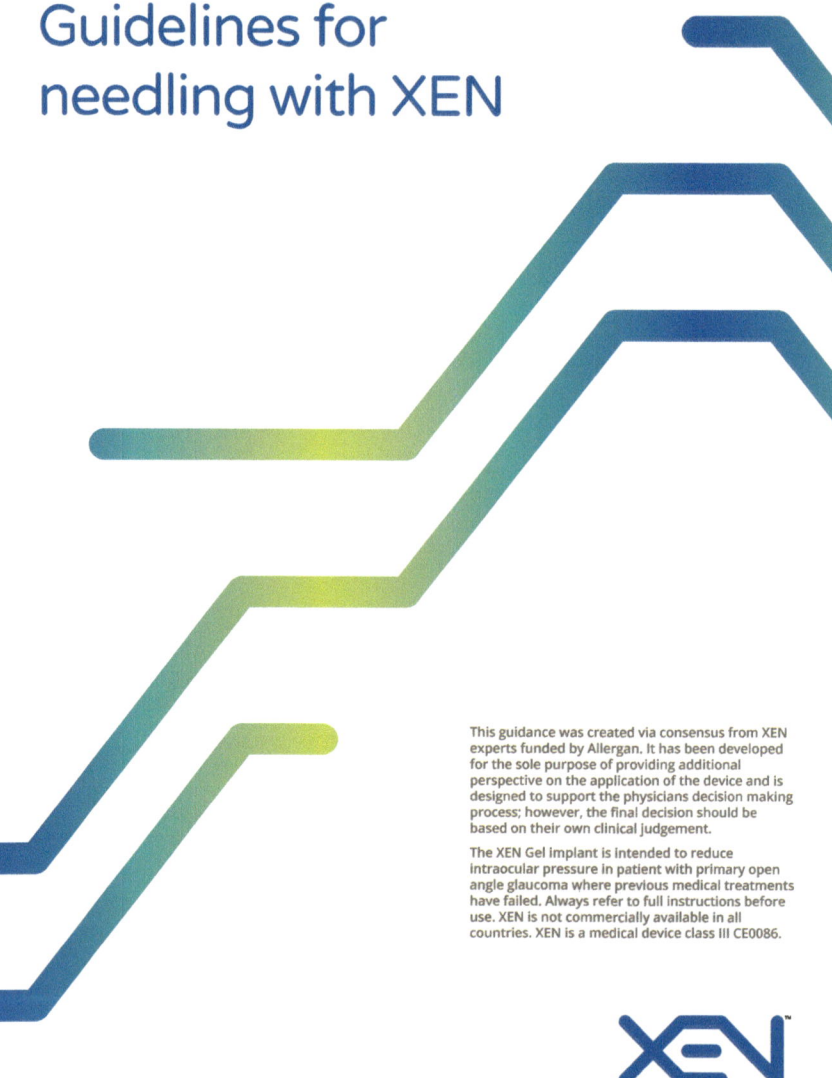

Guidelines for needling with XEN

This guidance was created via consensus from XEN experts funded by Allergan. It has been developed for the sole purpose of providing additional perspective on the application of the device and is designed to support the physicians decision making process; however, the final decision should be based on their own clinical judgement.

The XEN Gel implant is intended to reduce intraocular pressure in patient with primary open angle glaucoma where previous medical treatments have failed. Always refer to full instructions before use. XEN is not commercially available in all countries. XEN is a medical device class III CE0086.

XEN™

GLAUCOMA GEL IMPLANT

1   What is needling?

Following filtering glaucoma surgeries, wound healing processes may cause conjunctival remodelling which can decrease the efficiency of aqueous outflow of the bleb (resulting in a rise in intraocular pressure [IOP]). Needling is a secondary surgical procedure intended to restore aqueous outflow.[1] As with trabeculectomy, three types of XEN needling can be distinguished:[2]

Type 1:

Dissection of fibrosis in the subconjunctival-intraTenon's space[1]

Type 2:

Clearance of occlusions at the implant tip (analogous to scleral flap needling)[1]

Type 3:

Needling of a cystic (encapsulated) bleb if aqueous suppressant therapy proved unsuccessful[1,2]

All the above types of needling may be indicated to enhance aqueous outflow following XEN implantation. This necessitates a degree of skill in the evaluation and experience in the management of XEN post-operatively.

2   When is needling indicated?

Following three simple steps BEFORE choosing to needle may help improve post-operative decision making and avoid unnecessary interventions.

Step 1: Measure the IOP[2,3]		Justification for needling	
		Weaker	Stronger
IOP	Is IOP elevated (irrespective of bleb appearance)?	No	Yes
IOP vs target	Is IOP at/below target or above target?	At/below target IOP	Above target IOP
Change over time	Is IOP stable or has it increased since last follow-up?	Stable	Increased

Step 2: Rule out other causes[2,3]		Justification for needling	
		Weaker	Stronger
Steroid response	Is the patient using steroid medications?	Yes (consider steroid response if bleb is present)	No
Occlusion of the XEN internal ostium	Is the anterior chamber end of the implant occluded? (gonioscopy)	Yes (consider other rescue strategies)	No

Step 3: Assess the bleb and implant[2,3]		Justification for needling	
		Weaker	Stronger
Bleb appearance (slit lamp or OCT)	Is the bleb elevated? Are microcysts present?	Elevated bleb with microcysts present	Low, thick bleb without microcysts present
Response to digital ocular compression (DOC)	Is it possible to increase the size of the bleb following DOC? If so, how easily and to what extent?	Bleb size increase over a large area in response to modest DOC	No bleb size increase in response to considerable DOC
Mobility of implant	Is the tip of the implant still mobile (independently of the conjunctival tissue)?	Implant freely mobile independently of the surrounding conjunctiva	Implant fixed within conjunctival/Tenon's tissue
Mobility of the conjunctiva	Is the conjunctiva and Tenon's tissue mobile adjacent to the implant?	Tissues are mobile	Tissues are immobile
Bleb patency assessment (BPA)	How easily can the contents of the bleb be moved posteriorly? (using a blunt instrument or finger pressure on the eye lid)	Bleb contents can be easily dispersed posteriorly	Bleb contents cannot easily enter surrounding tissue
Visibility of the implant	Is the implant visible beneath the conjunctival tissue?	Implant obscured by opaque overlying tissues (consider revision)	Visible implant

4   Which instruments can be used?

	Application[2]
30-G needle	Useful for finer needling e.g. implant tip clearance (type 2 needling)
27-G needle	Larger cutting area useful for increasing bleb area mechanically (type 1 needling)
23/24-G MVR blade	Fine cutting edge useful for delicate tip clearance as well as increasing bleb area

5   How do I needle?

- Anticipate the risks for subconjunctival haemorrhage (e.g. patients receiving anti-platelet therapies, conjunctival hyperaemia) and prepare the patient/conjunctiva accordingly[2]
- Further minimise bleeding by avoiding blood vessels and using a vasoconstrictor[2]
- Plan your needle entry site and passage of needle movement before entering the subconjunctival space[2]
- Bending the needle/MVR blade at an angle aids access to the desired site and ease of rotating the cutting edge of the needle/blade[2]
- If appropriate, practice simple manipulations at the slit lamp[2]

- For simple needling cases, have preferred equipment available in clinic to avoid the need for rescheduling e.g. needles, anaesthetic, forceps, disposable speculum[2]
- During needling, agents which modulate the wound healing response may also be administered at the surgeon's discretion[2]
- Consider surgical revision if;[2]
  - Multiple attempts at needling have not sustained acceptable IOP, or where
  - The implant cannot be visualised due to a dense and opaque layer of Tenon's tissue

6   How do I know if I was successful?

Following 'successful' needling, decompression of the eye may be subtle (taking several minutes) and occur more slowly compared with a trabeculectomy needling. Confirming restoration of flow into the bleb can be enhanced in several ways, including:[2]

1. Digital ocular compression combined with bleb patency assessment (described previously)[2]
2. Achieving next day IOP <11mmHg may be indicative of long-term prognosis[4]
3. If unsure, intracameral administration of a vital dye can aid visualisation of restored aqueous flow and the size of the bleb area[2]

7   How should inflammation be controlled after needling?

Anti-inflammatory agents 4–6 times daily for 1 month and taper slowly over 2–3 months.[2]

References:

1. Feldman R. US Ophthalmic Review. 2011;4:26–8
2. Allergan Unpublished Data. Needling Basics, INT/0277/2018 May
3. Vera V, et al. US Ophthalmic Review. 2018;11:38–46
4. Broadway DC, et al. Ophthalmology. 2004 Apr;111(4):665-73

IOP, intraocular pressure; BPA, bleb patency assessment; DOC, digital ocular compression; G, gauge; MVR, microvitreoretinal; OCT, optical coherence tomography.

Adverse events should be reported to your local authority and your local Allergan office.

Allergan does not advocate the use of off-label medicine.

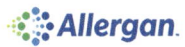

INT/0380/2018

eyecare
beyond now

Date of prep: June 2018

XEN Clinical Scenario Management Guidance

The following guidance applies to specific clinical scenarios relevant to XEN post-operative management. This guidance is intended to inform surgeons on the contributing factors and options for management.[1]

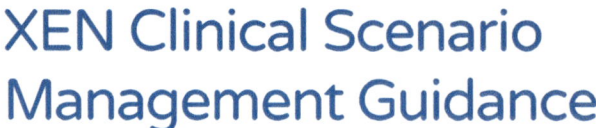

This guidance was created via consensus from XEN experts funded by Allergan. It has been developed for the sole purpose of providing additional perspective on the application of the device and is designed to support the physicians decision making process; however, the final decision should be based on their own clinical judgement.

The XEN Gel implant is intended to reduce intraocular pressure in patient with primary open angle glaucoma where previous medical treatments have failed. Always refer to full instructions before use. XEN is not commercially available in all countries. XEN is a medical device class III CE0086.

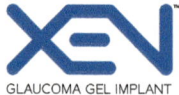

GLAUCOMA GEL IMPLANT

1   A large (mega-) bleb[1]

Presentation (may include):

- Corneal desiccation/epithelial defects/dellen
- Large (circumferential) and/or medially oriented bleb (**Figure 1**)
- Discomfort (dysaesthesia)
- Reduced best corrected visual acuity (BCVA)

Contributing factors:

- Nasal placement of XEN implant
- Over filtration e.g. due to short needle tract
- Female
- Body profile (overweight, loose skin, short neck)

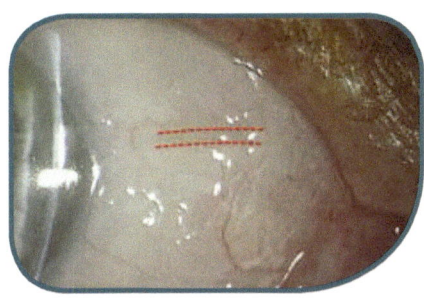

Figure 1 – Large, medially oriented bleb (red marks indicate XEN location). Courtesy of Herbert Reitsamer

Strategies for management

Objective: To create a more favourable bleb morphology that most commonly involves migrating the bleb in a more superior and/or posterior direction.

- Conventional bleb remodelling strategies[2,3]
  - Primary strategy: Aqueous suppressants
  - Secondary strategy: Compression sutures
  - Tertiary strategy: Electrocautery
- Surgical revision with/without diverting flow by a 'realignment suture' (**Figure 2**)
- Dry eye therapy
- If the implant is positioned very nasally, consider removing the XEN and implanting a second XEN close to the 12 o'clock position

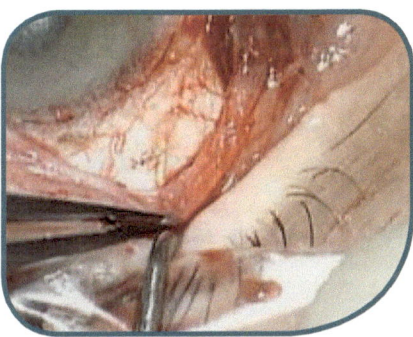

Figure 2 – Realignment suture.
Courtesy of Dan Lindfield

2   Erosion/leakage[1]

Presentation (may include):

- Implant exposure through the conjunctiva
- Seidel positive
- Low IOP (but not necessarily hypotonic)
- Epiphora

Contributing factors:

- Implants positioned in a location with high lid margin interaction e.g. scleral exit of the implant close to the limbus (short scleral channel)
- Implants positioned in a location not protected by the eyelid e.g. nasal placement

- Thin conjunctiva or Tenon's pre-operatively
- Ocular surface disease/dry eye
- Superficial placement of implant under the conjunctiva
- Short implant section in the subconjunctival space (results in tenting of the conjunctiva at the implant tip)
- Perforation of the conjunctiva with the XEN injector needle
- Post needling

Strategies for management

Objective: To close the defect in the conjunctiva. The approach may depend on the size and location of the defect.

- Depending on the cause of the defect (e.g. injector needle perforation), small leakages may resolve without intervention. An aqueous suppressant medication may further facilitate resolution

- Suture the defect (Buttonhole defects in the conjunctiva, for example those occurring with trabeculectomy, can be sutured[4]) (**Figure 3**)

- If the conjunctiva is fragile or the defect is large, consider revising the bleb to ensure the defect is fully closed when suturing

- Taper down steroids

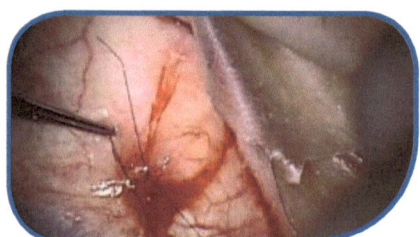

Figure 3 – Suturing conjunctival defect.
Courtesy of Herbert Reitsamer

- In rare instances, the implant may need to be removed to lower the risk of recurrence

3   Persistent hypotony[1]

Presentation (may include):

- Low IOP
- Choroidal effusion/detachment (**Figure 4**)
- Shallow anterior chamber
- Reduced visual acuity
- Maculopathy (**Figure 4**)
- Rarely, hypotony may result in more serious complications e.g. suprachoroidal haemorrhage or malignant glaucoma

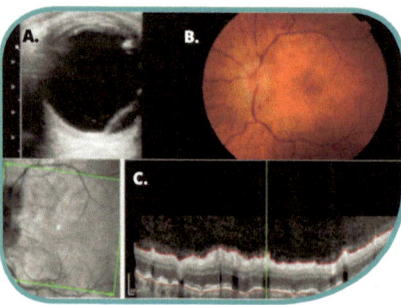

Figure 4 – **A.** UBM scan of choroidal detachment, **B.** Fundus image of hypotony maculopathy, **C.** OCT scan of hypotony maculopathy. Courtesy of Dan Lindfield

Contributing factors

- High refractive errors (high myopia)
- Low aqueous humour production e.g. post-cyclodestructive procedures
- Short scleral channel

- Cyclodialysis cleft (**Figure 5**. Typically as a result of a downward injector 'flick' during implantation)
- Filtration around the implant (unregulated outflow)

Strategies for management

- UBM imaging and/or gonioscopic evaluation to rule out cyclodialysis cleft
- Reduce steroid if over filtration is suspected
- Initiate short-acting cycloplegia if anterior chamber is shallow
- Refill the anterior chamber (0.10–0.15 ml) with dispersive viscoelastic if the anterior chamber is shallow or the visual acuity is reduced. Specifically avoid high molecular weight viscoelastic[5]
- In rare instances:
  - Bleb compression sutures may be required if the bleb is large
  - The implant may need to be removed if the IOP cannot be restored to a level where sequalae are adequately managed

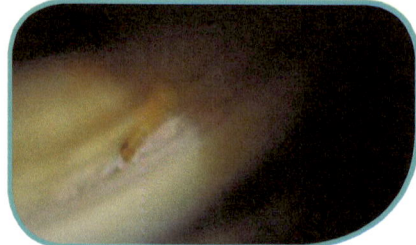

Figure 5 – Cyclodialysis cleft. Courtesy of Dan Lindfield

4 Avascular bleb[1]

Presentation (may include):

- Pale, thin, avascular bleb (**Figure 6**)
- Pain/discomfort
- Bleb leakage/oozing

Contributing factors

- Use of antifibrotic agents in glaucoma filtration surgery
  - Dosage too high for the wound healing propensity of the patient[6,7]
  - Dosage too high for the conjunctival status[6,7]
  - Repeated use of antifibrotics during intra-operative and post-operative management
  - Antifibrotic exposure to the limbal area of the conjunctiva[8]

Strategies for management

- Careful monitoring and observation[9]
- Dry eye therapies for discomfort or ocular surface abnormalities[10]
- In cases where there is a risk of blebitis, consider surgical excision of the avascular zone and placing healthy autologous conjunctiva over the bleb using either advancement of the conjunctiva or suturing a free conjunctival patch/amniotic membrane graft[9]
- Patients with symptoms and good IOP control should be evaluated carefully and informed that IOP may increase if a surgical re-intervention is chosen[9]

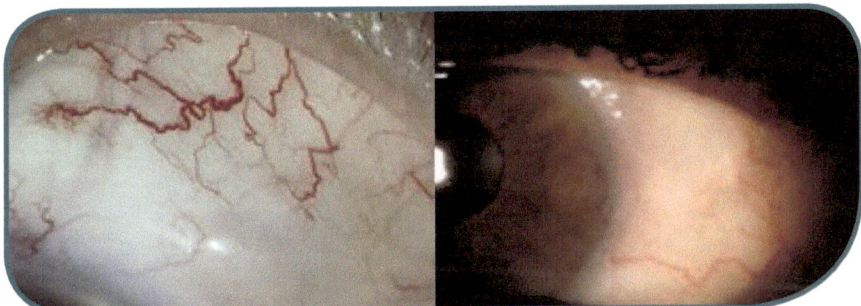

Figure 6 – Avascular bleb. Courtesy of Herbert Reitsamer

BCVA, best corrected visual acuity; OCT, optical coherence tomography; UBM, ultrasound biomicroscopy.

References:

1. Allergan Unpublished Data. XEN Clinical Scenario Management Guidance, INT/0276/2018 May 2018
2. Lloyd M, et al. Arch Ophthalmol. 2008;126:1759–64
3. Al-Aswad, L. Glaucoma Today. 2006. Available from: http://glaucomatoday.com/2006/06/0506_03.html/. Accessed May 2018
4. Vijaya L, et al. Indian J Ophthalmol. 2011;59:S131–S140
5. Bruynseels A, et al. J Glaucoma. 2018;27:e75–e76
6. Habash A, et al. Clin Ophthalmol. 2015;9:1945–51
7. Vera V, et al. US Ophthalmic Review. 2018;11:38–46
8. Anand N, et al. Br J Ophthalmol. 2006;92:175–80
9. Budenz, D. Bleb Leaks. Glaucoma Today, 2009;October:33–35
10. Sagara H, et al. Eye (Lond). 2008;22:507–14

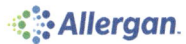

INT/0379/2018

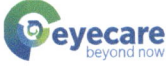

Date of prep: June 2018

Appendix G: PRESERFLO MicroShunt Glaucoma Device Surgical Technique

Narrative Instructions By Santen Pharmaceutical Co. Ltd.

Authors: Omar Sadruddin MD, Yasushi Kato PhD
Raymund Angeles MD, Leonard Pinchuk PhD.

The PRESERFLO MicroShunt Glaucoma Device is intended for placement through a transscleral *ab-externo* approach allowing the proximal end of the device to be placed in the anterior chamber while the distal end of the device is placed under the conjunctiva/sub-Tenon's capsule.

The following description of the procedure is not a substitute for the comprehensive surgeon training provided by Santen to new users. The surgical steps and technique for the PRESERFLO MicroShunt Glaucoma Device are as follows:

Preparation of PRESERFLO MicroShunt

Carefully examine the package containing the PRESERFLO MicroShunt for signs of damage that could compromise sterility. If damaged, discard the device. Remove the PRESERFLO MicroShunt from sterile packaging onto sterile field. Wet the PRESERFLO MicroShunt using a solution of Balanced Salt Solution (BSS).

1. **Anesthesia:** The type of anesthesia will be at the surgeon's discretion (e.g., subconjunctival). Standard ophthalmic surgery techniques according to institution protocol should be used to prepare the patient and the eye for surgery

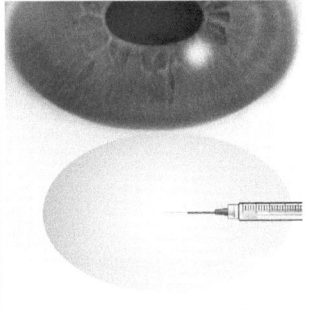

2. **Corneal traction and subconjunctival flap:** The use of corneal traction with 7–0 suture (e.g., Vicryl or silk) will be at the surgeon's discretion. Dissect a fornix-based subconjunctival/sub-Tenon's flap at the superonasal or superotemporal quadrant over a circumference of 90–120° at least 8–10 mm posterior to the limbus. Use cautery, if necessary, to achieve hemostasis for a bloodless field

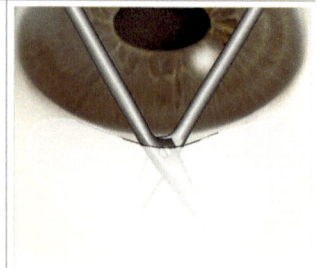

3. **Application of mitomycin C (MMC):** Apply sponges saturated with 0.2–0.4 mg/mL MMC to the surgical site for 2–3 min

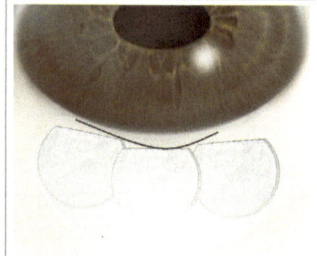

4. **Rinse out Mitomycin C:** Remove the sponges from the eye and copiously irrigate the surgical site with balanced salt solution (>20 mL)

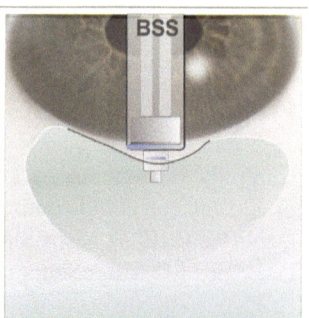

5. **Preparation of anterior chamber entrance site:** Using the ruler provided in the PRESERFLO MicroShunt kit, after being inked with the gentian blue pen, mark a point 3 mm from the posterior border of the surgical limbus (blue/gray zone)

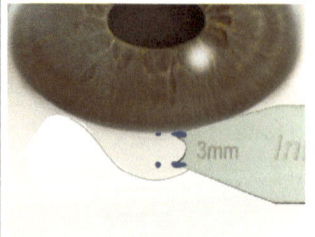

6. **Incise scleral pocket:** At the distal marked point on the sclera, use the provided 1-mm wide disposable slit angle knife to create a shallow scleral pocket, 1–2 mm long to tuck the fin portion of the PRESERFLO MicroShunt

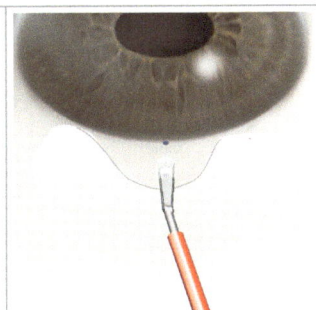

7. **Create 25G needle tract:** Maneuver the 25 GA needle tip, bevel up, into the apex of the scleral pocket and create a transscleral tract into the anterior chamber. The scleral track's entrance into the anterior chamber should bisect the angle just above the iris plane with sufficient clearance from the posterior cornea

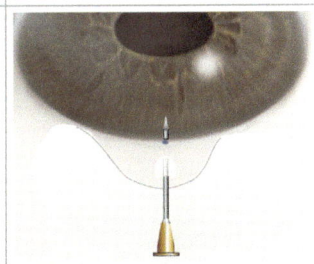

8. **Insertion of the PRESERFLO MicroShunt into the anterior chamber:** With a pair of forceps, hold the promixal end of the PRESERFLO MicroShunt, bevel up, 1 mm from tip. Thread the PRESERFLO MicroShunt gently into the transscleral tract at approximately 1-mm increments, to prevent kinking, until the promixal tip is in the anterior chamber. If difficulty is encountered during the insertion of the PRESERFLO MicroShunt into the anterior chamber, consider creating another transscleral tract approximately 1–3 mm to either side of the original one. A new PRESERFLO MicroShunt may be necessary if the previous one was damaged during the initial insertion procedure

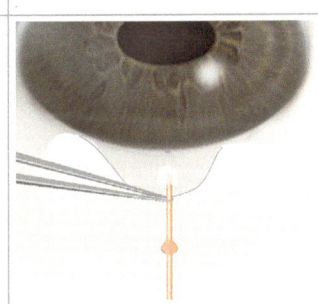

9. **Insertion of the fin into the scleral pocket:** After successful insertion of the PRESERFLO MicroShunt into the anterior chamber, wedge the fin into the scleral pocket. Ensure that the PRESERFLO MicroShunt is not in contact with the iris and the posterior part of the cornea.

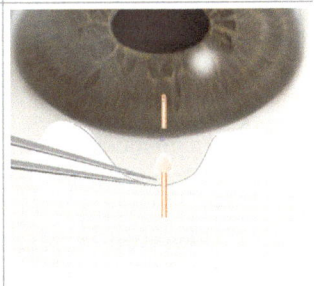

10. **Confirm flow:** Confirm consistent percolation of aqueous humor at the distal end of the PRESERFLO MicroShunt. Slight pressure on the cornea will help initiate flow. If flow is not clearly visible in the form of percolation or a slowly growing bead of aqueous humor, consider using a 23 GA cannula attached to a syringe filled with balanced salt solution to prime the PRESERFLO MicroShunt. It may also be necessary to create a paracentesis to reform the anterior chamber.

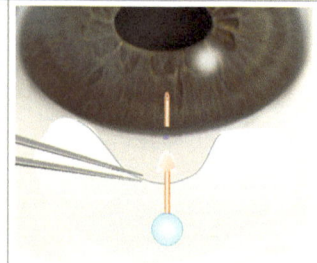

11. **Tuck PRESERFLO MicroShunt under Tenon's capsule:** Once flow is established, tuck the distal end of the PRESERFLO MicroShunt underneath Tenon's and conjunctiva, making sure that it is straight and free of tissue

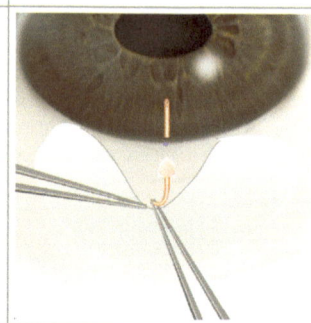

12. **Conjunctival closure:** Reposition the Tenon's and conjunctiva to the limbus and perform closure using sutures with a well-established history of successful use in glaucoma surgery (e.g., Nylon, Vicryl). Consider suturing Tenons first and separately to avoid any retraction postoperatively, followed by closure of the conjunctiva. Use a moistened fluorescein strip to check for leakage from the wound or from conjunctival tears. Additional suturing may be necessary to control leakage. Verify that the proximal end of the PRESERFLO MicroShunt is in the anterior chamber and that the distal end is straight. Remove the corneal traction suture if used

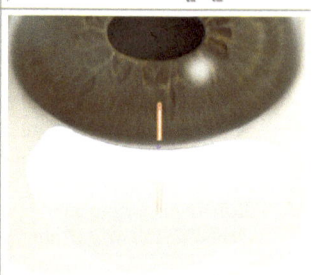

Note: No cutting or modification of the PRESERFLO MicroShunt is recommended.

Postoperatively:

1. Apply antibiotic and steroid medication postoperatively according to usual practice for trabeculectomy.
2. Monitor the intraocular pressure at each standard-of-care follow-up to determine if the PRESERFLO MicroShunt is functioning.
3. If the PRESERFLO MicroShunt is repositioned, removed, and/or replaced with another type of device or another PRESERFLO MicroShunt, due to lack of efficacy, the conjunctiva should be cut at the limbus in a similar manner to the original implantation procedure. The PRESERFLO MicroShunt should be exposed and the repositioning or removal conducted thereafter. After the PRESERFLO MicroShunt is removed, verify that there is no aqueous leakage from the transscleral tract. Suturing of the transscleral tract with Vicryl will be necessary if leakage is detected.